Thriving in Adulthood

with

Asperger's Syndrome

by

Craig Kendall

Sign up for Craig's free
Asperger's Syndrome Newsletter at

www.AspergersSociety.org

First published in 2010
by Visions Research
PO Box 1257
Solana Beach, CA 92075
Copyright 2010 by Visions Research

www.VisionsResearch.com

Printed in the United States of America
ISBN 978-0-9841103-2-2

2

Dear Reader,

I want to thank the readers of my newsletters who have written to me over the years and told me they needed this book; and to those who helped me make this book a reality. I receive hundreds of emails per week asking for advice. I tell everybody the same thing—I am not a therapist—I am a parent who has struggled for nearly two decades to understand Asperger's syndrome. I give my suggestions and advice, my Asperger's Chicken Soup, which comes primarily from you, the tens of thousands of you who have lived through it, and found your way.

Over this period I have often turned to you for answers, the many subscribers to my Asperger's Syndrome Newsletter. And you have consistently responded through countless surveys, helpful emails, and heartfelt stories.

And this book is no different. In this book, I have asked my newsletter subscribers to share with me their personal lives. Their stories. Their successes. Their failures. What it feels like to have Asperger's syndrome. And I received many emails. I cannot print all the emails I received or this book would be too heavy to lift. But I have selected a representative sample to bring to life the reality of Asperger's syndrome. I especially want to thank those who shared their stories.

Craig Kendall

Table of Contents

Asperger's is not a curse—it is just a difference, and a difference that can be worked around.

Introduction

I've decided to start this book with a story. A story from an adult with Asperger's syndrome. My purpose in choosing this particular story is that if represents a *realistic* look at how life can be for an adult with Asperger's. It is not "white washed" and polished. It does not say that life is a bed or roses—for those with Asperger's know that life is often challenging. But it also shows that Asperger's brings many benefits as well as challenges. Throughout this book, I share stories of courage, struggles, success—and yes, failure. You CAN live a happy rewarding and successful life with Asperger's, filled with friends and loving, nurturing relationships. For some, it is a long journey. Hopefully, this book is a roadmap on how to get there.

Dave's Story

2009 was the year I turned 45. It was also the year I was diagnosed as having Asperger's syndrome. My response was none of the clichéd ponderings over why this was my lot, or how could it have happened or even how cruel and cavalier life can be. Rather, I felt an oddly relaxing sense of peace. Finally, so many of my life experiences made so much sense. It made me happy to understand at last.

I already knew about Asperger's as my brother has it. His is, apparently, a more severe case than mine. Further, I previously worked with people with disabilities and came across Asperger's in that work. I am a curious sort of person (read that anyway you like), and so I have researched the condition extensively. I understand it. The diagnosis has helped me to understand so many things about myself. It makes sense of why I struggle to multitask. Why I had episodes that I now know are my 'meltdowns'. My mind cannot process information in quite the same way as other people, and so I become "choked up" and anxious.

Meltdowns also happened when people bothered me for favors. Now I know why I have a bad history of caving into favors. Why I feel such a doormat. I learned in childhood that giving into the demands of others (reasonable and unreasonable alike) has been a way of reducing the meltdown pressure. That pressure is distressing in ways I can only barely describe.

Meltdown pressure is chaos and mayhem wrapped in headaches and confusion. It feels like drowning in a deathly sea of turmoil and guilt and anguish. A meltdown is the mental equivalent of choking on a cob of corn; only there is no one around to give me the Heimlich maneuver. My meltdowns are, I believe, on the way out of my life, as I am adopting strategies to manage them. I use meditation and thought-stopping techniques and these are already melting my meltdowns away.

Like a lot of Aspies (as we affectionately call ourselves) I am also a survivor of abuses by others. It seems this "disability" is characterized by the possession of too much empathy. We tend to care "too much" for others. Yes, contrary to what some would say, many Aspies are afflicted by a condition in which we actually do care for

11

our fellow creatures. Whether they have fins, wings, fangs, four legs or two, as an Aspie, I care about them. I wish only love and peace to all creatures. It is why I follow a vegan diet and wear leather-free shoes (even though they hurt my feet). Yet in having such loving thoughts for my fellow creatures, I have, too often, been too naïve to notice the darkness behind some people's thoughts and actions.

Sarcasm eludes me. I mentally understand what it is, and can even exercise it with some effort, but I find it very hard to detect it when it is being wielded against me. This has made me the butt of many jokes. I am saddened by the fact that so many people I love are filled with such sadness. I am even more saddened to realize that the universal love I hold for others is regarded as a symptom of a disorder.

Is love really a disorder? Is vision? What about imagination, compassion and the capacity to concentrate on one task, to do it well and to see it to the very end, no matter what it takes?

All of these traits describe Asperger's syndrome. Yes, there is sadness involved; sadness and difficulties and privations. Yet most of these are caused by the neurotypical world's lack of imagination, compassion and poor concentration skills.

I am glad I am blessed with this syndrome. I think my life would not have been quite so pained, nor anywhere near as interestingly rewarding, had I been afflicted by a neurotypical mind. This is truly a case of the good outweighing the bad. Asperger's means I have an unwavering ability to ignore social convention and seriously question the truth behind so many harmful things that are taken as givens by most upon this cold, blue world of ours. That is a wonderful trait for a writer (or indeed any artist) to possess. Yet there are genuine negatives.

Relationships are where it hurts the most. Asperger's has created so many misunderstandings and so much loneliness in my life. It has also meant so very much heartache, depression, abuse, psychosis and worse. Yet now, I am very fortunate to have an amazing lady in my life. To find someone so patient and understanding is one of the biggest blessings of my life. I also have many very good friends and colleagues. I am able to help care for my ailing parents, whom I love dearly.

I know this all makes me so very lucky. I also know it means that I must have a lot of awfully good karma banked up.

So G'day, my name is Dave.

I am a boyfriend. I am a son. I am a brother. I am an uncle. I am a friend. I am an Australian. I am a writer. I am a dreamer. I am a colleague. I am a student. I am a teacher. I am a pain. I am a benefactor. I am a klutz. I am an Aspie. I am lucky.

I am happy.

Above all, I am happy.

Dave

***

1. Surviving the Social World: How Do You Make and Keep Friendships in Your 30s, 40s, and Beyond?

Welcome to your guide about life with Asperger's syndrome as an adult. You are probably aware that there are a large number of guides and books written for parents of kids with autism and Asperger's; they cover almost every possible topic. There might be a few written for teenagers and young adults. But where does that leave the older generation? Those who came of age many years before Asperger's was even an official diagnosis in the psych manuals? The ones that grew up knowing something was different about them and being shunned for it—but having no idea what and why.

You might have survived most of your life on coping skills you developed and honed yourself but by the time you get to middle age, you're probably getting pretty tired of it. You want to stop struggling so much. You want to be able to make friends without so much effort. You want to be able to hold down a job, date, and feel good about your life. But no matter how much you try, you keep failing; it seems like no one will even give you the time of day. Everyone thinks you're weird; no girl or guy will return your phone calls when you ask for a date; your boss keeps giving you the pink slip, no matter what the job.

This guide is for you.

To start, we are going to talk about some ways that you can start to make, and keep friends.

Part One: Making and Keeping Friends

The basic issues of difficulty with socialization and friendship have been covered extensively in the media and most material on Asperger's. We will review it briefly here for anyone new to the topic.

Social deficits are a major problem in Asperger's syndrome (AS). People with AS are often very bright, but lack social savvy. They miss social cues. They don't understand nonverbal language. They take everything very literally. They are tied to routine and exactness.

Sometimes they talk in a rather pedantic style. You can usually tell an Aspie—an affectionate term for those with Asperger's—as they are the ones that will be standing to the side, looking a little out of place, talking about details that no one else thought of, worrying about things that no one else thought to worry about, and coming up with facts and knowledge about the situation that no one else knew. Aspie adults kind of march to the beat of their own drum. And, quite often, they have a very hard time matching and recognizing the beat of someone else's drum.

There is a famous joke about how to identify an Aspie that I will share with you.

> A guy is flying in a hot air balloon, and he's lost. He lowers himself over a field and calls to a guy "Can you tell me where I am and where I'm headed?"

> "Sure. You're at 41 degrees 2 minutes and 14 seconds North, 144 degrees 4 minutes and 19 seconds East; you're at an altitude of 762 meters above sea level, and right now you're hovering, but you were on a vector of 234 degrees at 12 meters per second."

"Amazing! Thanks! By the way, do you have Asperger's syndrome?"

"I do! How did you know that?"

"Because everything you said is true, it's much more detail than I need, and you told me in a way that's no use to me at all."

"Huh. Are you a clinical psychologist?"

"I am, but how the heck did you know that???!!??"

"You don't know where you are. You don't know where you're going. You got where you are by blowing hot air. You put labels on people after asking a few questions, and you're in exactly the same spot you were 5 minutes ago, but now, somehow, it's my fault!"

When this joke was told to a group of people with Asperger's they first laughed and said it was very accurate. Then, two people tried to look up the exact coordinates of the place given in the joke to see where it was located. That is just another example of the detail oriented, fact loving nature of many people with Asperger's.

All digs against clinical psychologists aside, the joke has a point. The Aspie will always be the one who gives far more detail than is needed, knows all kinds of facts, but can't seem to present them in a way that seems coherent at all.

Aspies tend to have very strong and narrow interests. Adults with AS also fall into this pattern. They are very into trains, or a particular baseball team, or World War II history, or music—it could be anything. They may try to talk to their co-workers or potential friends excessively about these things. They may not look at their co-workers or friends in the eye; they may appear to be quite anxious.

Anxiety is an unfortunate turn-off for many people. When so-called "typical people" interact with someone with AS, the anxiety and nervousness that so many with Asperger's have often makes the typical person uncomfortable. Often, the person with AS has no idea what signals they are sending.

The DSM-V (Diagnostic and Statistical Manual of Mental Disorders), which is the handbook for all psychological disorders, has this to say about social communication impairment in their official criteria of Asperger's:

"Qualitative impairment in social interaction, as manifested by at least two of the following:

1. marked impairments in the use of multiple nonverbal behaviors such as eye-to-eye gaze, facial expression, body postures, and gestures to regulate social interaction

2. failure to develop peer relationships appropriate to developmental level

3. a lack of spontaneous seeking to share enjoyment, interests, or achievements with other people (e.g. by a lack of showing, bringing, or pointing out objects of interest to other people)

4. lack of social or emotional reciprocity."

Basically, it means problems using all of the many social skills that come naturally to most people in order to engage in and maintain conversations and relationships with other people.

Here are some other social gaffes and deficits that might get adults with AS into trouble socially:

1. Not realizing when someone is trying to change the subject, or end the conversation, when talking to them.

2. Not remembering to ask questions about how the other person is doing and to take an interest in them.

3. Lack of eye contact, awkward body postures, fidgeting, inappropriate facial expressions, lack of knowledge of how to use nonverbal communication.

4. Not seeming to understand or be sensitive to others' feelings, or at least not showing this understanding in a recognizable way.

5. Not being able to "read" other people well, and having trouble understanding or using humor.

6. Tone of voice: either speaking in a monotone, or not being able to modify your tone of voice to fit the situation.

7. Sensory issues: may have trouble paying attention and focusing on communication due to loud noises in the environment, too much visual chaos, the feel of touching something uncomfortable (such as wearing uncomfortable clothes), unpleasant smells, etc. Easily distracted.

8. Conversation often sounds stilted and unnatural. Since most Aspies need to almost "go off a script" to figure out what to say in any given social situation, it is going to sound somewhat rehearsed and unnatural, because it is. Aspies are at a great disadvantage because no matter how much you practice, and try to learn what to say and how to say it, it's hard to make it sound natural—you are speaking a foreign language, after all. This will often turn off others who feel uncomfortable with

the forcedness of it. People seem to sometimes instinctively turn away if it seems like you're "trying too hard." Non-Aspies want to engage in easy, seamless conversation; they want to let off steam and shoot the breeze; they don't want to have to put much effort into what they're doing (not all typical people, of course, but this fits many), and when they encounter someone who seems to "not fit in" to their conversational model, it makes them want to seek easier conversations. They might engage you for a few minutes and try to be nice but there is usually a limit to how long they will accommodate someone else's conversational difficulties.

9. Problems maintaining a friendship—many Aspies do not realize that once you make a friend, you have to do things to maintain the friendship. You have to initiate phone calls, schedule outings, inquire as to the other's well being, and so on. You can't just drop off the face of the earth and show up when you feel like it.

Sounds daunting, huh? With all of these difficulties, it's amazing that adults or anyone with Asperger's even attempt any conversations at all. Communicating can be like speaking a different language for people with AS.

Margot Nelles, founder of the Asperger's Society of Ontario, describes the experience of Asperger's in the following way: "It's like being dropped in the middle of rural China without a guidebook or a language book, and you go from home to home and feel that somehow you have insulted everyone."

Most people with Asperger's who have been told of that quote agree very much with the experience. They talk frequently of the experience of trying to follow the social rules and put themselves out there, to chat up their fellow co-workers or people they meet, but being unable to understand why the response is so negative. Since they don't read social cues well and since they just naturally appear to be on a different wavelength, a lot of people just don't get them—and a lot of people don't want to take the time to try to understand.

This is not to say every single person will reject a person with Asperger's on first contact! There are a lot of lovely people with compassionate souls in this world. They understand what it is like to be different and think differently and they have patience, understanding and the desire to understand people who present differently. These are wonderful people who should be sought out as much as possible; but unfortunately, there are not as many of them in the world as there should be, and they can often be hard to find.

The experience of trying to make friends as an adult with Asperger's can be lonely, isolating, and discouraging. Adults with AS try, try, and try again but get continuously rebuffed and sometimes do not have enough insight into, or understanding of, their condition to understand why. So they do not know what to change or they do not know how to change. Or, sometimes, they believe they do not need to change; that people should just accept them the way they are. So they face continuous rejection by making the same mistakes over and over again. It can be depressing.

When you leave college and high school, the opportunity for making friends out of your peer group and fellow students, as hard as that is, goes away. Isolated in an apartment, it is hard for even typical people to go out and make friends. But it is much harder for those with AS. The best thing to do is to find friends out of interest groups or meet others with AS too, as will be discussed later on, but some adults have too much anxiety and insecurity to be able to do this. They are afraid they will be judged. They are just afraid to go out. Sometimes, they will go to groups

if they have a friend or family member go with them—
sometimes not.

Experiences of Friendships from Adults with AS

Listening to the stories of what adults with AS have to say
about their difficulties in making and keeping friends can
give us a lot of insight into the situation. Many adults with
AS are very open about their difficulties. Below is a
sampling of some things that actual adults with Asperger's
have said about making friends. Most were found on
Internet discussion groups for people with AS, such as
WrongPlanet.net.

An Aspie by the name of GreenPele reports that he can
make friends but he can never seem to keep them.

> "The problem for me is not making friends. I mean I'm
> not like my brother who makes 5 or 10 life friends every
> time he goes to school, but I do start a friendship with a
> couple of people at school or on forums. The problem is
> that they never stay my friends for long. Usually after
> several months they kind of get "bored" with me, and
> everything I say irritates them or drives them away. And
> then when I ask if I'm boring them or if they're too busy
> they always get annoyed. Then one day we just stop
> talking or seeing each other completely.
>
> Now I may not be a Social Butterfly, but I do require
> people to talk to when I get bored or lonely, and it just
> frustrates me that I can't keep friends for long. In a way
> it's caused me to not trust people, because when I do
> make a "friend", I always know the friendship won't last
> forever. I bet a lot of other people feel this way too?"

Another user, Seanmw, agreed and tried to understand why
his friendships never seemed to last.

> "Yeah, my friendships always turn out to be "unstable",
> eventually they all seem to fray at the edges and fall
> apart of their own accord.

I guess it's because I'm not very entertaining. I can pull off that kind of charade for maybe a month or so before I run out of material to work with. And they tend to lose interest in me. And so drift away like the superficial beings they are. I found one or two friends however that, while not being Aspies or on the spectrum as far as I know, don't like small talk just like me and we get along okay. Though the guy's a freaking chick magnet (has beautiful hair and is a musician, go figure) and so the jealousy's there."

One person says that friendships tend to go downhill for him quickly because few people understand his needs. People with Asperger's tend to have many needs that the average population either doesn't understand or doesn't want to deal with; sensory issues such as sensitivity to loud music, lots of chaos, fragrances, and so on; they need structure and routine, need to plan ahead, desire to avoid large crowds, etc. This can make them seem rather undesirable to other people as the other people often do not want to spend a lot of time trying to meet the needs of the person with AS, and decide often that it is better just leaving them alone.

ActiveButOdd says,

"I have trouble keeping friends. I can attract people and have them like me to a point, but things go downhill from there.

The people may expect me to handle more than I can deal with, like expecting me to eat in a restaurant or cope with seeing a movie, or travel around rapidly somewhere I don't know well/at all, deal with crowds etc. They may become over familiar, talking/touching too much, asking personal questions, wanting 'more', or merely being someone I can't seem to handle.

People don't seem to get me and the different challenges I face. This means they won't understand the way I behave, and I may be judged or labeled as being/acting a certain way when it has come about through something I am experiencing."

Adults with Asperger's will often try very hard to fit in with their peers. They will go to bars and try to "shoot the breeze", so to speak. Bars and clubs are a major place of socialization for many Americans; and, in many workplaces it's almost expected that you will gather at the local bar after work to bond. This type of interaction is not a normal, natural thing for most Aspies. Bars are very loud places, very distracting to be in, and difficult places to have conversations. And the quality of conversations in a bar is usually very low. Aspies tend to like more intelligent, thought-provoking conversations—so fitting into a bar atmosphere is really not a good idea for them. But nevertheless, they try. And sometimes become rather depressed at the results, which often makes them hesitant to try again—in any venue.

One member of Wrong Planet, Acacia, had an experience very similar to this. He reports:

"I get to the bar last night, meet up with them. We have a drink, things are fine. Of course, I'm in sensory-overload-anxiety-panic-mode... but I'm hanging in there, and the alcohol helps. Then it all starts to go downhill. By the second drink, these guys are getting loud, cursing up a storm, talking in a really graphic way about all the things they've ever done to women, and all the crazy stuff that they did/destroyed/regretted when they were drunk. And this kind of talk just didn't stop.

I would try and talk about something interesting, or creative, or... you know, thoughtful. They actually looked away from me! They didn't pay attention to the things I said, and seemed like they couldn't care less.

This went on for a couple of hours, and I kept trying to figure out a way to leave. I didn't want to be rude, considering this was supposed to be some kind of cool reunion thing. But all it did was make me a wreck of anxiety and completely uncomfortable. Eventually, I paid my tab and said I had to go. They gave me strange looks of confusion as I got away from that place as quickly as I could.

Today I just reflected on how utterly ironically terrible this all was. I actually got out of the house and attempted to be social with my peers! And it was profoundly disturbing."

The experience of being the only one in a group wanting to talk about thoughtful, more intelligent subjects is an experience very, very common with Aspies. They just don't do small talk well. They don't understand the meaning of "shooting the breeze"—conversation needs to be structured and meaningful. This works for some people; there are people out there who do not have AS and still want to have intelligent conversations. A lot of them, even. But you have to look pretty hard for them, and you have to know the right places to find them.

Part Two: Where Can Adults with Asperger's Find Friends?

Okay, so if you've read this far, you know WHY adults with Asperger's have trouble making friends—and if you are an adult with Asperger's, this is probably sounding pretty familiar by now! But let's now talk about ways to solve all of the problems outlined above.

Yes, it is hard to make friends if you are an adult with AS. Yes, it's lonely. But there ARE things that can help. There are organizations that can help; and tools and strategies that can help. Let's talk about some of them.

Local Asperger's Support Groups

The first line of defense, so to speak, for adults wanting to make friends should be Asperger's groups and organizations dedicated to such things. This is because Aspies will tend to get along better with other Aspies as a general rule. It is wonderful to meet other people who think the same way you do, act the same way you do, talk the same way, and just generally understand you. Now, there is diversity in the Aspie population just like in the rest of the world. You won't automatically get along with every Aspie in the world, but you do have a much, much better chance. You can find someone who shares your interests, someone who wants to "be" and interact in the same way that you want to.

Many of these organizations run support groups for adults with Asperger's—some can put you in touch with others with AS.

Find a Group in Your City

Many cities have their own Asperger's groups and meetings. These are definitely worth finding. Washington, DC, for example has a very large group called "Asperger Adults of Greater Washington," or AAGW. It has almost forty people come to meetings every month. Most groups are not nearly that big. They meet in one corner of a tea cafe once a month. At the beginning, they have social time for their members to talk with each other—then they sometimes have a speaker or a discussion topic, and more free form social time at the end.

Every group for Aspies is run differently. Some focus on just free time for conversation, some are all speakers, some discussion based, some are more therapy oriented. Some only have as few as 4 members; others, like AAGW, could have as many as forty.

The wonderful thing about these groups is people are usually very nonjudgmental. You can feel safe there, safe to be yourself. If you fidget a lot and can't look anyone in the eyes, no one will care. If you talk about trains all day, they will understand. If you have too much anxiety to talk but just want to sit and listen, they will be glad to have you there. Whatever your level of functioning and way of being in the world, at an Aspie group you will be greeted sincerely. Most people are very friendly, although of course it depends on the person and group; and you will feel welcome. You will recognize yourself in others. You will feel less alone.

The OASIS website maintains a great list of local support groups in all fifty states. A lot of these are for parents but there are some for adults with AS too. This is located at http://www.udel.edu/bkirby/asperger/

Also, try using Google to find local groups, or email a national Asperger's email group to ask if anyone there knows of local groups (Examples are grasp.org groups, ASAN at http://www.autisticadvocacy.org/, Autistic Daily living Yahoo group, etc.)

National Asperger's Advocacy Groups

In addition to all the local groups, there are a few national or regional Asperger's organizations that run support groups for adults with Asperger's. These are all very useful groups to know about.

GRASP, or the Global and Regional Autistic Self Advocacy Network, runs support groups for adults in several different states but focuses on the New York City region. Their current list of support groups include locations in California, Colorado, Iowa, Illinois, Michigan, New Mexico, Pennsylvania, Virginia, New York and more. There are several based in the New York City area. GRASP's website is located at www.grasp.org if you wish to learn more.

ASAN, or the Autistic Self Advocacy Network, runs groups in several different states as well. These are run by

26

people on the autism spectrum and are often focused more on political issues (such as advocating for rights for people on the spectrum, and how to work to reduce the number of negative messages about people with autism in the media, how to educate people about autism spectrum disorders, etc.).

ASAN's website talks more about the goals of the organization. It was started by two young men in their 20s, both with Asperger's. One was just starting college, one in grad school; both with a vision to create an organization for people with autism spectrum disorders; An organization run by people who had the same disorder in order to create a welcoming place of support and also to create an organization that would fight for the rights of people on the spectrum.

ASAN describes its mission the following way on their website's mission statement, located at: http://www.autisticadvocacy.org.

> "The Autistic Self Advocacy Network seeks to advance the principles of the disability rights movement in the world of autism. Drawing on the principles of the cross-disability community on issues such as inclusive education, community living supports and others, ASAN seeks to organize the community of Autistic adults and youth to have our voices heard in the national conversation about us. In addition, ASAN seeks to advance the idea of neurological diversity, putting forward the concept that the goal of autism advocacy should not be a world without Autistic people. Instead, it should be a world in which Autistic people enjoy the same access, rights and opportunities as all other citizens. Working in fields such as public policy, media representation, research and systems change, ASAN hopes to empower Autistic people across the world to take control of their own lives and the future of our common community. Nothing About Us, Without Us!

The Autistic Self-Advocacy Network (ASAN) is a non-profit organization run by and for autistic people. ASAN's supporters include autistic adults and youth, those with other distinct neurological types and neurotypical family members, professionals, educators and friends. ASAN was created to provide support and services to individuals on the autism spectrum while working to change public perception and combat misinformation by educating communities about persons on the autism spectrum. Our activities include public policy advocacy, community engagement to encourage inclusion and respect for neurodiversity, quality of life oriented research and the development of autistic cultural activities and other opportunities for autistic people to engage with others on the spectrum."

A third organization is the Asperger's Association of New England, or AANE. They provide support groups in most of the six New England states. They are based in Boston, and have several groups in that area. They have social activity groups, where members go to various places together (bowling, out to dinner, to see a lecture), as well as support groups and social skills groups. A full listing of groups can be found at www.aane.org.

A great website to find support organizations and support groups which lists groups broken down by U.S. state is: www.aspergersyndrome.org

The listing of support organizations here is extensive. While these listings are not necessarily all oriented for adults, with a little work, you can likely find a support group that will meet your needs.

How Else Can Adults with Asperger's Find Friends?

It's useful to meet other adults with Asperger's, but sometimes you just want to be able to make friends with the people around you. How can you accomplish that? How can you develop more friendships in your life?

> ## Work on your social skills

One option is always to get counseling to help work on your social skills. A good counselor can tell you where you're going wrong and work with you to help change the weak areas. They can identify those areas in which you need help, and model proper social skills. They can role model with you what to do and say in social situations. By working with a skilled therapist, you can be more aware of the way you come across, and gain more friends with your new, improved skills.

> ## Seek out people you are compatible with!

But you still need a place to meet the right people. All the social skills in the world aren't going to help you get along with just anyone. People have very different personalities, interests, and communication styles. You need to meet people who are compatible with you.

But how do I do that, you ask? Well, look around you. Decide what you have an interest in. If you like to read, join a book club. In the process of discussing the Great Gatsby, you just might stumble upon a kindred soul. Like to swim? Join a swimming club. **Many Aspies make friends much better when they are DOING something with a person instead of just talking to them**. They need something constructive to do while being with a person; that way the focus is on the activity instead of the conversation.

If you like history and World War II, join a historical preservation group. Maybe you can get involved in Civil War reenactments.

If you're into sports at all, join a sports club; non-competitive sports are probably more likely to spur friendships than competitive, but you never know. If you like to sing, join a choir. If you like to write, find a writing group. The list is endless. The important thing is to match your skills and interests to a group of like minded people. You might still have social skill issues, but you'll have a common interest with these people and be much more likely to develop friendships. Just be patient and know that developing friendships takes time; it doesn't happen overnight. Go slow and try not to rush things. Trying to rush into things will put pressure on the other person and make them much more likely to end the burgeoning friendship prematurely. It is hard to wait, yes, but worth it in the end.

Eight Places to Find Potential Friends

1. Intellectual interest groups

Book clubs, political discussion groups, moral and ethical discussion groups such as Socrates Cafe, MENSA are all good places to look.

2. Athletic Pursuits

Look into local groups for soccer, basketball, swimming, or any sport that you have an interest in.

3. Creative Activities

Arts and crafts, photography, painting, writing, and other creative arts; people meet to share work, discuss technique, or engage in said art during group time with others.

4. Religious Organizations

Churches and synagogues can be great places to meet others. Often they hold their own discussion groups, choirs and activities.

5. University Groups

If you have a college or university near you, they may hold special interest groups that are open to the public that you could join.

6. Science and Technology

Do you like computers? Science fiction? Medicine? Find like-minded people in a group dedicated to these topics.

7. Your Workplace

Sometimes you can find like-minded people in your workplace, or at least people to go out to a baseball game with. A lot of times this doesn't happen, but it can occasionally.

8. Activity Groups

People might meet to play board games, chess, Scrabble, go hiking, or do any manner of activity together.

But how do I find these groups?

Lots of ideas, yes, but they can be hard to find in real life. The first thing you should do is check your local newspaper to see what is listed. Usually there is a calendar that lists all the activities, entertainment and groups that will be meeting that week. Independent, free weekly newspapers often tend to have longer and more comprehensive calendars of this nature.

Go to websites like www.Meetup.com and Craigslist.com to look up groups in your area. These websites can be wonderful resources for social connections.

www.Meetup.com lists any and all of a wide variety of interests groups in your area. From knitting to photography to Scrabble, they have it all; just put in your zip code. CraigsList.com has a smaller selection usually but can have interesting social opportunities under their Groups section.

Where to Find Interest Groups

- Your local newspaper

- Independent, free weekly newspapers

- Craigslist.com

- www.Meetup.com

The Internet

If you are too nervous or have too much difficulty making friends in person, you can try support groups on the Internet. There can be amazing benefits in participating in online support groups as well as local ones. For one thing, they are a lot easier to find. If there is nothing available locally, an online group can be a wonderful support.

For another, the anonymity of writing online can be freeing and easier to communicate with for some. Many people can communicate better in writing than they can in person. Many people with Asperger's who get very nervous in social situations where they have to look people in the eye and decipher body language flourish online where the only thing that matters is the words that you write, not the body language that you use to convey them in. Additionally, when you connect to an online group, you have an amazing wealth of resources at your fingertips. You can meet people from all over the world, and learn so much from the accumulated knowledge of all the people who are participating. You can pick up tips and gain emotional support in much the same way you would do face-to-face.

One great resource for Asperger's support online is www.wrongplanet.net. There are other online resources as well. Try to find interest groups online by doing Google searches. You may be able to find local people to be friends with by meeting them on Internet sites dedicated to an interest you have.

There are also email groups, the most popular of these being Yahoo groups (http://groups.yahoo.com). With a Yahoo email group, you subscribe to a particular group and get emails from other people who have also subscribed. You can read their messages and reply.

There is an abundance of Yahoo groups for autism spectrum issues—one need only to search the site for "autism" or "aspergers" to find them.

Tips for Interacting with People

Well, now you know where to find people, and how to find people, but what do you do when you meet them? How do you make a good first impression? Here are some tips.

1. **Be aware of your body language**. Try to look at people directly, or at least in their general direction. Try to smile. Try to speak slowly and clearly. Try not to fidget too much. If you have trouble looking people in the eye, here is a trick you can use—look at the end of their nose. You may find this more comfortable and they will never notice!

2. **Ask them about themselves**. Don't focus the conversation on yourself too much. Don't talk about your special interests. Try to find an area of common interest. Comment about the event you are both at, or about the weather, or some issue of

current events. Avoid any heavy, emotional or controversial topics.

3. **Pay attention to social cues**. If they seem to be getting bored or irritated, stop talking. Wait for them to talk. Make sure to acknowledge what they said before talking about your own stuff again. Keep your replies somewhat short. Graciously end the conversation if the other person seems to be getting irritable or seems like they want to leave. There will be other opportunities for conversation with this person in the future.

4. **If you see them again, make sure to be friendly**. Say "Hi" and "How are you?" If phone numbers were exchanged, make sure to follow-up and call the person.

5. **If the other person seems amenable, suggest an activity you would both enjoy doing together**. Make sure it is something the other person would enjoy too!

6. **Above all, be patient**. Just because you don't hit it off with one person doesn't mean you won't with anyone. Keep trying. Ask for feedback from someone you trust if you suspect your behavior or presentation is turning people off. Take new friendships slowly. You will find someone you connect with before too long if you follow these rules.

What Not to Do to Find and Make Friends as an Aspie

As mentioned before, it is very important to choose the right kind of places to hang around to try to make friends. Some adults with Asperger's will get depressed when they go to a party and can't interact with anyone there. They can't keep up with the conversations, they don't know what to say, they feel very left out. Everyone seems to ignore them and they can't figure out why.

Well, it turns out, there are certain social arenas that have some pretty definite (but hard to understand) social rules that Aspies are usually not equipped to figure out. And in areas like this, they suffer because of it. An advice column called "Dear Aspie" on WrongPlanet.net very deftly addresses this issue and explains why it is an issue at all:

> "Among Aspies, there's a myth that goes something like this: "NTs (Neurologically Typicals) socialize because they gain glorious, heartfelt relationships that fulfill them and bring them warmth and joy." Well, go say that to an NT. You'll get roars of laughter. So why do NTs indulge in so much mingling and sparkling, chatting and joking?
>
> The important point to understand is that socialization is by and large a game for NTs. You're an Aspie, so you're likely unaware of it, but when you go into a party full of laughing, drinking people, you're actually stepping onto a gigantic chessboard. On this board, NTs are competing for mates and sex, social position, admiration, money, power, and just about anything else you can think up.
>
> Most NTs love the game of socialization. Not only that, they assume everyone else does, too, so they don't think of it as offensive to play the game with one another. Moreover, they are so deep into the game that few are aware of it. Therefore, much of the socialization you see hides maneuvers, and it's neither genuine nor lasting. Now, we Aspies don't see our way in this game clearly, if at all. That's why Aspies can't stand parties, and why the myth arises. We walk into a room of smiling, laughing people, and we put ourselves in their positions: "Boy, if I were laughing and talking with somebody like that, I'd feel great. I'd feel sincere and connected." Then we assume that NTs feel that way, too. (But they don't.)

35

Now, to tackle your problem: can Aspies have real friendships and relationships? Yes, they can. But you're not going to find them in the usual places. Friendships need a basis. If you go to parties and sit around the keg trying to base your friendships or loves on playing the socialization game, you will almost certainly be smashed and ignored.

But there are alternatives. Sports is a good example. Or, if you're not athletic, bird watching clubs, chess clubs, church food drives, dancing lessons, collecting clubs … and the list goes on. The important point: these activities place you on the same team as the people you're sharing space with, not in social competition with them. And in these activities, you're much more likely to run into someone who's looking for someone just like you. Those people (from your past) likely demanded moves of you that you didn't comprehend. When you didn't respond as required, you seemed hopeless to them."

This is a hard lesson for those with Asperger's to learn: some social communication has no real purpose at all. It is a kind of jockeying for position. It has rules they will probably never understand. It is this kind of social interaction that Aspie adults should probably try to stay away from, if they are looking for success at making friends. **Interest groups are great; bars and parties, not so great—at least if you want to make long lasting connections.**

Final Words

In conclusion, there are many reasons why adults with Asperger's have so much trouble making and keeping friends. They don't understand social cues; they have sensory issues that prevent them from functioning well in some environments; they have different ways of talking and communicating that are not well understood by many, and they have anxiety issues, among other things. But there are also many ways to overcome these issues: attending groups for people with Asperger's and meeting people there; and attending a wide variety of special interest groups where they can meet like minded people. Paying more attention to how they present themselves can help increase chances of success. If you follow the advice in this chapter, you or your loved one will be well on their way to increased social success.

2. Asperger's and Relationships

Relationships. What a tricky thing, huh? There are probably few things in this world more difficult and complicated to navigate than a relationship with another human being.

Even people without Asperger's have plenty of difficulty with this one. Reading other people's signals, showing explicitly that you care for them, figuring out how to get your own needs met while meeting the needs of the other person, figuring out how to work together—it can be an Asperger's nightmare!

Unfortunately, nearly all of the skills that one needs to make a relationship work are also the skills with which people with Asperger's have the most difficulties. People with Asperger's often have trouble reading nonverbal messages, explaining their feelings explicitly, anticipating others' needs without being told explicitly, and so on. But does this mean that relationships are doomed—for both people with AS and those who love them? Of course not! It just requires a lot of education for both parties to learn how to work effectively together. This chapter will attempt to help you navigate this complicated path—it is written for both people with AS looking for relationships, and people who love those with AS and want to make their relationships work better.

Open a newspaper, turn on the TV or look at a magazine stand. Everywhere, everyday, we are bombarded with messages about relationships. "Ten Tips to a Sexier You!" "How To Improve Your Relationship in Ten Minutes," and so on. Stories about celebrity relationships. Stories of relationships gone horribly wrong. It is no secret this is something many people covet. In fact, sometimes it seems the world revolves around people breaking up and getting together. People want to feel loved; to feel a sense of belonging; to have a sense of fitting somewhere. They want to feel cared for and appreciated by others. They want someone to share their bad days and to celebrate their triumphs. Relationships with others, both romantic and sexual, are a big part of the way our world works.

This importance, however, can make it very lonely for those who, for whatever reason, can't seem to find themselves in a relationship. Yes, everyone wants to feel loved, but what do you do when you can't seem to master the social skills necessary to find and keep a relationship? What if you never get past square one? What if you can't even say hi to a member of the opposite sex, or at least make it past a first date without making a complete fool out of yourself? This is a problem many with Asperger's have. It can leave them feeling very lonely and isolated. They want to be a part of the dating world; and being left out can cause bitterness, resentment, and depression. Even those in relationships are often unhappy because things are going wrong in the relationship and they don't know how to fix them.

Six Steps to Building Successful Relationships

There are many challenges for adults with Asperger's in developing successful relationships—as well as for their partners. In order for relationships to work, an adult with Asperger's must learn to overcome the deficits in their social skills tool set. They must learn the rules of relationships.

Generally speaking, those with Asperger's are highly intelligent, they want deep meaningful relationships—but are frustrated and bewildered about how to get them. By the time AS adults are in their 20s, 30s, 40s, 50s or older, many are very set in their ways and some have given up trying. But there is hope. By focusing on the following six issues, an AS adult can gain the tools needed to have successful relationships.

1. Reading Social Cues

People with Asperger's have a lot of difficulty reading and understanding social cues. They have difficulty with nonverbal language. They have difficulty with the "give and take" of most conversations and interactions. So, this means if a woman has a "come hither" expression on her face and wants her partner to do one thing, the AS partner might completely miss it and comment on the sports scores in the newspaper, or talk about the strike going on in town. Or if one partner is angry and wants an apology but doesn't come out and say anything, the AS partner will often be completely unaware that anything is wrong.

Someone with AS may not be able to look at your face and your body language and get any information from it. You often need to be very explicit in the messages you give an AS person for them to understand. This can be very frustrating to both people.

People with AS often don't understand social norms. For example, they may not understand that you have to engage in casual "social chit chat" or small talk with someone you have just met before getting into anything deeper. You need to get to know each other before asking that person out on a date. You shouldn't tell your life story to someone five minutes after you've met them. You shouldn't tell a woman she has a pimple or smells, even if she does, if you want to preserve the relationship—at least not at the beginning of a relationship—and probably not ever!

These are all things that are common sense for most people, but not for people with AS. The AS adult might go up to a woman he likes and ask her out immediately without bothering to get to know her, or he may do other things "out of order," or have a sense of intensity about him that feels uncomfortable to the other person. For this reason, it is often hard for the person with AS to get past saying hello when trying to find a potential date or partner. There is a lot of social etiquette that is beyond the reach and knowledge of most people with AS. This doesn't make them lesser people or not worth getting to know by any means but just like in a job interview, it can make it hard for them to even get a chance.

2. Showing Emotions, or Picking up on Emotions

People with AS often show emotions in very different ways than do their NT counterparts. Many people with AS have trouble showing their emotions at all. They may feel very bad about something that has happened, but be unable to say "I'm sorry," or "I feel bad about what I did." This can lead to anger and resentment on the part of the other person.

Some people with AS show emotions inappropriately; for example, laughing during a serious moment or a conflict. Some are over-emotional and let too many emotions come out and this can overwhelm the other person. Emotional regulation is a difficulty. A person with AS might likely have trouble controlling their anxiety when they are worried or uncomfortable, might yell or cry very easily and so on. Both sides of the spectrum are represented when it comes to emotions. Some Aspies might not even be aware of what they feel, and others might be overwhelmed by what they feel but not know how to process it, or communicate it very easily.

Most people with AS have trouble reading the emotions of others and responding to them. So they might not know you

41

are sad or upset just by looking at you as most people would. But they can learn—they can learn to figure it out by asking questions about how their partner's day went and by inferring from the answers a possible emotional state. For example, if you went to the dentist you might not be feeling very well, but if you went to a friend's birthday party you likely are feeling pretty well. This can't always be assumed, but it is a start.

Many non-AS partners of people with AS become frustrated when people with AS fail to respond to their emotional state. We all want people to make us feel better if we are down in the dumps, and to celebrate with us when we have had something good happen. If AS is involved, it is important to try not to take it personally if your partner—whether you are dating or in a permanent relationship—does not seem to be responding in the way you would like. Try to give more explicit clues to your state. Say "I am feeling X," or even, "I am feeling X and I would like you to do Y for me."

Many adults with Asperger's want to help very much but often have no idea how or what is expected of them. For adults with Asperger's, try to ask questions about how your partner's day went, and imagine what they might need from you—or simply ask them! You will probably get a much better response that way. This is not something that comes intuitively, but it can be learned; one can do it manually.

3. Being Flexible

Flexibility is a big one. People with AS have trouble with mental flexibility. They have a mental map and a plan for how they will do everything. This gives them a feeling of security. Without this base of security to work off of, they are lost. They flounder. They cannot tolerate uncertainty and have difficulty with change.

However, in a relationship, things come up that have to be accommodated. If you have to take someone to the doctor at 8:00 am, your husband might need to re-arrange his schedule and get up earlier than usual to watch the other kid. Or if you are running late and need someone to start dinner, or go to the pharmacy to pick up a prescription because you're not able to, and your AS husband hadn't planned to do this, he might have trouble re-arranging his schedule in his mind (even if he is not doing anything specific that would prevent him from doing these things) in order to do them. If you usually have movie nights on Friday night, but one night you want to watch a movie on a Thursday, this might cause discomfort. If you usually have dinner at 7 but one night have to wait until 9 or have it at 5, this may be a problem. Or if you want to order from a different place, or if your husband needs to cook when you usually do... These are all examples of flexibility that, to different degrees, people with AS can have a lot of trouble with. This can be a big hindrance on a relationship, because it hinders the smoothness, the "give and take" and flow of a relationship.

Mental flexibility is another issue, or perhaps part of the same one. Even in conversations, sometimes, a person with AS will be following a script of what they think they "should" say and will have trouble deviating. When people with AS attempt to flirt, it often comes out sounding unnatural and forced—it is hard for people with AS to think or do things on the "spur of the moment." This makes them come off as somewhat weird and makes it harder for them to attract and interest potential mates.

While it is good to have a sense of routine, people with AS need to figure out a way to be prepared for deviations in their schedule when things come up. They need to be willing to do things out of the norm of what they would usually do, to the best of their ability, if they want to be able to keep a healthy and satisfied relationship with another person. Therapy can help with this and sometimes just time and working on it gradually with a supportive partner can help a person improve his or her abilities in this area.

4. Taking Someone Else's Perspective

This is a big one for people with AS. It is often called "theory of mind." People with AS often have trouble imagining where someone else is coming from. They have trouble imagining that someone else could see the world from a different vantage point than they do or have different opinions and ideas than they do. In short, taking someone else's perspective. This can be frustrating both for the person with AS and for the other person in a relationship. The AS person genuinely wants to understand where the other person is coming from but often just can't. And many, of course, are not aware that they don't understand in the first place—they are blinded by their own perspective.

For example, if you ask your AS spouse to help clean up the house he—or it could be she, but we will use he just as an example—replies, "Why? It's not dirty." He is not necessarily trying to be obstinate, but to him it genuinely does not look dirty and to clean it would seem a waste of time and energy that could be better spent elsewhere. He doesn't understand that a) this is something important to you, and that is reason enough to do it, and of course b) different people have different ideas of levels of cleanliness. Or, if you suggest, "Let's go to the movies and see *Tuscon Bridges*," a movie you have wanted to see, and he says, "I heard that got awful reviews, and I hate love stories. I don't want to go," he may not understand that sometimes, not always but sometimes, you do things you don't want to do to make the other person happy.

He can only see what he wants to do. This is something that can cause a bit of a strain on relationships. Taking the perspective of another person is a necessary part of being able to understand and respond to that person, of being able to care for them. The partner can feel a sense of resentment. It is important, then, for the person with AS to try to realize that his or hers is not the only perspective.

When your partner asks you to do something or if you want to do something, stop for a minute. Think. Why does he or she really want me to do this? Would this be something that would help her in some way? Would it hurt me more than I can handle to do it? If not, then consider doing it—or work out a plan of how often you will do this thing, and when, if not at that particular moment. Show your partner you care about his or her feelings and desires as well as your own.

5. Communicating Effectively

People with AS need everything to be explicit and blunt in order to understand. So if you want someone with AS to, for example, bring you breakfast in bed, you have to say, "Gee honey, it would be really nice if you brought me breakfast in bed Saturday morning, do you think you could do that?" He will probably be eager to help but wouldn't have thought of it otherwise. Or if you need help cleaning the kitchen, or you are frustrated with him for coming home late every night without calling, anything you might be thinking—you need to get in the practice of saying it, because he won't pick up on it otherwise. Even if it's something he's done before, if it's not part of his daily routine, it probably won't be in the front of his mind unless you say something.

People with AS speak in a very literal way, and don't read between the lines well. They don't play games or understand games others are playing. This can leave them hurt or unable to effectively communicate what they need to say. Misunderstandings are common. Both people need to make a conscious effort to talk out conflicts that arise before they get too big.

One member, Lisabee, contributed to an online Asperger's discussion site at www.psychforums.com by saying, "Quite often my husband and I will have a disagreement or he will be upset with me for not responding in the right way. He either wants more emotion or less emotion or a different response or something. Often times I just cannot work him out or work out what he wants. At those times he gets very annoyed with my response even though I have explained to him what I am meaning. I know this is related to having AS because the responses are that I am not showing enough emotion, or I say yes but with no tone in my voice and it is this which he doesn't like." This is related to the problems showing emotions and talking about emotions that we have discussed before, and is a common issue for adults with AS.

6. Dealing with Physical Contact and Sensory Issues

Some adults with AS don't like to be touched or hugged, at least not by people they don't know very well and sometimes even then. This makes the start of relationships sometimes uncomfortable and difficult.

Due to sensory issues many adults with AS have trouble going to places where one might often meet potential mates, such as bars, clubs, parties, and so on; these places are too noisy with too much chaos for them to be able to think or focus. They may wear clothes that are not exactly in style due to tactile sensitivities. They might be picky about what they eat or where. They may get overwhelmed easily.

For some, these issues cannot be overcome. In this case, it is better to avoid these uncomfortable situations, if possible. Instead of going to a noisy bar, find a quiet coffee shop for a date or get-together. If you are meeting family members, perhaps you can meet them in two or three separate gatherings, each with fewer people so that you feel less overwhelmed. If having a dinner with people at a restaurant pushes you over the edge, perhaps you can invite people to your home and cook for them. If you are more in control of the situation—being in your own home—you might feel more comfortable. And if you are cooking you can ask others to help out in small ways; peel carrots, open a bottle of wine, set the table. Many times it is easier for an AS adult to engage with others through activities, even simple activities such as helping out in the kitchen, than sitting at a large table in a noisy restaurant and trying to carry on a conversation about topics in which you have no interest.

User EvilKimEvil added to the discussion on issues she's had in relationships on a different Asperger's discussion group, www.wrongplanet.net. She has experienced many social misunderstandings due to her Asperger's. "My social issues have caused problems. I've had boyfriends get angry at me for wanting to leave a social event too soon after arriving, or not talking enough. They say, "You don't like my friends!", "Stop being so unfriendly!", "Why are you being rude?", "Relax. My family won't hurt you," etc.... And of course there have been issues with my tone of voice. I'll ask a benign question and it will be taken as sarcastic or complaining. This still happens all the time, but my bf doesn't make a big deal of it—I think he sort of understands." Kim's examples of being misunderstood are also common for many who have AS.

Relationship Tips for Asperger's Adults

Now that you know some of the ways that people with AS can be challenged in relationships, it's time to talk about some of the ways those with Asperger's can work around these issues—and, similarly, ways neurotypicals or NTs (a label for people who are not on the autism spectrum) can try to accommodate the Aspies in their lives.

Love is a two way street

Just because the person with AS is the one with challenges does not mean everything is "their fault." If you fell in love with someone in a wheelchair, you wouldn't think much of opening doors for them or providing some physical assistance to them—you'd do it because you loved them. It's just another part of them. Just the same, someone with AS has certain aspects that need to be accommodated and these aspects should never be looked upon as something that are "their fault." Both people in an AS-NT relationship need to work equally hard to understand and accommodate the other person. (Sometimes Aspies will date and have relationships with other Aspies; this is in many ways easier because a lot of the communication challenges are not present. For now, however, we will focus on AS-NT relationships.)

Tips for Aspies in Relationships with NT Partners

1. Engage the other person

Don't just sit there on the computer and ignore him or her. Make time for them. Remember why you love them. Make an effort to watch their favorite TV shows with them; to have conversations; to go out to places they like to eat. It doesn't have to be all the time, but make a conscious effort to engage them.

2. Make an effort

Make an effort to go to social events with your partner, if that is what they desire. Try not to refuse to attend due to discomfort; at least not all the time. Many people like to go out to dinners with friends or other events with their spouses; try to agree on how often this will happen.

3. Be more flexible

If you usually do something at a certain time, like have dinner or watch a certain TV show, and it doesn't happen that way one day, try to work around it. Try to be able to do things in a different way when the situation calls for it. Try to look at things in a different way. Your partner will appreciate you all the more for it.

4. Be attentive to and sensitive to your partner's needs

Try to realize when he or she needs some extra attention; when they need help with something around the house; or they just need peace and quiet—this goes a long way in every relationship. But sometimes Aspies have to work harder to realize what these needs are in the first place. Ask if you don't know. Say, "Is there anything I can do to help you?"

5. Surprise your partner with a kind gesture

Try to be spontaneous occasionally, and surprise your partner. Surprise them with flowers, chocolates, a note, anything just to say you were thinking of them. Do little things like that once in a while and it will increase the morale of the relationship. People like to know their loved ones are thinking of them.

Tips for NTs in Relationships with Aspies

1. Try to understand where the Aspie is coming from

His or her mind works differently from yours. They are not trying to be stubborn, rude or obstinate. Their understanding of things is just different. Ask questions to try to understand their way of thinking.

2. Be aware of an Aspies' need for down time

Be aware of the need that Aspies have for "decompressing" time; that is, they need breaks from the social world. They need time to themselves to let off steam. They need a lot of time to process what is going on around them, and what they have just done. Adults with AS will become overwhelmed by doing too much at once. Break large activities into smaller steps with time out in between.

3. Understand and overlook their social quirks

Understand that an adult with AS has many social quirks. They are likely not being rude if they leave in the middle of a conversation to take a break or speak in a blunt way. If they don't dress up to go out, it may be because of sensory issues. If they don't respond in the way you expect, they may not understand how they are supposed to respond. **Again, ask probing questions to figure out why they are doing what they are doing**.

Realize that many adults with AS have many sensory issues. If they are in a noisy, crowded, busy social setting, they may get overwhelmed. If they snap at you or someone else, they may be overloaded and need to leave. There is usually a reason behind the behavior.

4. Be explicit

Aspies need to be told things explicitly to understand them. If you want them to clean up the kitchen, don't hint at how messy the kitchen is; ask, "Would you mind sweeping the floor?" Subtleties are lost on most Aspies.

If you want them to be romantic, you might have to spell it out.

5. Plan ahead

Try to have a plan or routine for most things you do. Try to have things as spelled out, and as planned ahead of time as possible. This will make your Aspie partner feel much more at ease. Most Aspies hate it when you tell them 10 minutes beforehand on a Tuesday night, "Get ready! We're going to the theatre in ten minutes, and you're coming with me!" That won't work. If you want your Aspie partner to do something with you, ask them about it well ahead of time. Tell them, "Is it okay with you if we go to the theatre next Tuesday night to see a show?" If you want to go out to dinner, try to ask ahead of time. Try not to do things spur of the moment.

Jeff Deutsch, who writes the blog Common Ground at www.buildingcommonground.blogspot.com, has this to say about Aspie/NT relationships, and how he has worked to make his work:

"I've worked to accommodate Emily as an NT. I engage her as much as I have energy for, including watching a few of her favorite shows with her (often on DVD) such as The Sopranos and vintage episodes of Saturday Night Live.

I go to some events with Emily as a couple. Events which I've agreed to ahead of time with full knowledge of what's going on and who will be there. I make sure to get plenty of sleep the night before (a good night's sleep is like topping off the social fuel tank, especially—but not only—for an Aspie or autist), and I stay civil to everyone. If I sense my social fuel gauge creeping too close to the E, I leave and take a walk.

Meanwhile, Emily understands my nature…probably better than anyone else. She understands how I need to spend time decompressing by myself in front of my PC. She knows that I do enjoy conversing with her but often in 5-10 minute segments, often on predetermined subjects. When I ask her questions, she tries her best to give me answers that are direct, to the point and whenever applicable (e.g., how long, how soon, how much, how often) have a number in them.

We could both do better, and we're working on it. I'm working on reducing the time I spend with my PC to spend with her instead, and on going out with Emily more as a couple. Meanwhile, she knows that she needs to cut out her cracks about my employment and job search and her angry outbursts about my bluntness."

Jeff knows the true value of accommodation, and works hard to accommodate his partner, while she works to understand and accommodate him. Together, they have built a relationship that works for, and benefits, both of them. They are an example and testament to the fact that Aspies can indeed have successful relationships with other people.

Relationships with Other Aspies

Well, there is more than one way to approach this relationship thing, of course. While, statistically speaking, it may be easier to seek a relationship with an NT because there are more of them, it might also be to your advantage to seek out a relationship with another Aspie. There are many advantages and benefits to this. For one, you have a much better chance of understanding each other. You understand why the other person is sometimes stand-offish, why they need their downtime, and so on. You are more likely to communicate on the same wavelength. You might have similar quirks. There are fewer struggles in trying to understand the other person and gain acceptance. The flip side to the coin, however, is that each other person may have sensory or other needs that are sometimes incompatible. For example, one person might be really light sensitive and prefer to be in darkness most of the time, while the other person simply can't function without a lot of lights. One person might be really sensitive to fragrances, while the other person can't live without their scented lotions. It may take extra work to learn how to be flexible and share space with another person when both people are likely to be very rigid about their rules. These are things that come up in every relationship, but perhaps just more so when you have two Aspies together. But it can be done, and is worth trying if you have the opportunity.

Jerry and Mary Newport are one such example of a successful Aspie-Aspie relationship. There is a movie based on their life called *Mozart and the Whale*. Both grew up socially awkward, knowing they were different but not knowing why. When they found each other, they found in each other someone who could appreciate their weird and eccentric interests, someone who could take delight in the things only they would. According to an article by Kim Kowsky from the Los Angeles Times, "Against the Odds: A Love Story," from October 1995,

"Jerry recalls feeling instantly at ease with Mary. She was the first woman he had ever met who didn't make him feel self-conscious. 'We could do silly things together, like reading billboards backward and guessing what it said," he said. "Or I would turn license plate numbers into dates. Like if I saw the number 20,013, I could tell you that Oct. 17, 1955, is the 20,013th day of the century.' Mary was charmed by his mathematical abilities: 'I liked it. It was a different version of what I could do with my music and art.'"(Los Angeles Times)

There were also difficulties as well, of course. Since it is so hard for people with AS to read what others are feeling, and since it is sometimes hard to communicate about these things, the Newports had to work extra hard to understand each others' emotions and not take them personally when conflicts arose.

"Mary had to learn not to take it personally when Jerry shrank from her touch in pain. He had to learn to keep his voice down during disagreements to keep her from "emotional shutdowns" that render her speechless." (Los Angeles Times)

The Newports found each other at a Halloween party, where he came dressed as a whale, and she as Mozart. They met at a support group for people with Asperger's that Jerry had started.

There were some bumps in the road, and one divorce, but they eventually realized that they were better together than apart, problems and all.

Some people are of the opinion that shared interests are one of the most important things in a relationship. One Aspie writes on her blog, Veiled Glory, on wordpress.com that, "What keeps us together and happy is having many interests in common. This might seem like common sense to everyone, but for Aspies/Auties, I believe this is a crucial element of a close relationship. We thrive in our special fascinations. If my interest were sewing quilts and Jeff's interests had nothing to do with fabric, we would be hard pressed to share time together. Our respective accouterments of interests would compete for space (uuhhh, it already does, but still). We would get testy. Those small threads of commonality might break. Ugly.

Aspies also use their special interests to communicate with the world. If you both speak a different "interest language", you might have difficulties in other parts of your marriage. We have quite a bit in common and some things that are not."

She goes on to list some of the things they have in common: the Christian faith, museums, computers, baking, hiking and growing plants. Common interests can be a great starting point for a relationship.

Aspies often feel more comfortable with others when they are physically doing something, as in sharing an activity, rather than just talking, so all the better to share an interest together. When an Aspie is with another person and they are just talking, sometimes there is a lot of pressure to think of things to say, and it can be stressful to try to fill the space. Sharing an activity, like bowling or hiking or going to a lecture together, gives you something to do with each other naturally. That is why special interests groups can be a great place to meet potential partners.

How to Meet Others

The first step to finding a relationship, of course, is to try to find a partner. This is hard for many people, not just those with AS. In our modern life, we are very isolated. In the past, there were arranged marriages and family had more of a say on whom you got together with, but for most cases, that is not true anymore. So how do you find that special someone? Well, it is different for everyone; but there are some places, it goes without saying, that are better to look at than others.

Some environments are better than others

If you have AS, there are some environments you are going to do better in than others. So, for example, hanging out in smoky bars to attract mates is probably not for you. The music is too loud, the conversation too superficial for most, there is nothing of substance going on—and Aspies usually like to meet people who they can have conversations of substance with. So, it might be a better idea to go to art gallery openings, book clubs, or college lectures if you're hoping to find a more intellectual type.

Find groups centered around your interests

Figure out what your interests are, and follow them. Try to find groups centered around those topics. Science fiction clubs, chess clubs, public speaking, archery, you name it. The first step to a good relationship is often having something in common. Of course, if you go to these groups expecting only to find a mate, you will probably be disappointed. These things take time, and you will scare away any potential dates if you seem desperate or like you are pressuring someone. But if you put yourself into situations where this kind of thing is more likely to happen, eventually you might get lucky and find someone you hit it off with.

What about online dating sites?

There are also dating sites online, which many people have had success with. The great thing about online dating sites is it allows you to find someone who might share similar interests and have things in common with you, without having to search endlessly for them. It is like looking through an encyclopedia of possibilities and having a computer sort them out for you. Many dating sites charge a fee to use. You email potential matches, and if they like you, they email you back. There are many different kinds of sites like this, the biggest probably being Match.com. Some dating websites are even geared specifically to Aspies, like www.aspieaffection.com. Some sites, like Plenty of Fish (www.plentyoffish.com) are free of charge and feature a very simple, easy to use interface.

User Jxenu, discussing Aspie dating websites on the website Aspies for Freedom (www.aspiesforfreedom.com), says about his experience with online dating sites, "I think dating sites can be very useful for many Aspies. You get to know someone before meeting them in person, so the typical Aspie social oafishness doesn't really get a chance of chasing off someone you are interested in but don't know. By the time you meet them in person, the other person knows your good qualities and likely already knows you're socially awkward.

Take me for example. I really couldn't get a date the "usual" way to save my life. But I've had 3 significant online relationships, and all three of the ladies wanted to marry me at some point, so I guess there is something good about me. (I actually did marry the last one) I believe the two others were also Aspies. Like everything else, however, it's not for everyone."

One final idea on potential places to find dates: you could try something like speed dating; in this event, you rotate through a series of potential matches and get to spend about seven minutes each with them. It is not ideal for Aspies who like more in depth conversation, but it's better and more well-organized than a bar scene.

What Not To Do On a First Date

Okay, well you've done it, you found a potential match. You're on the first date. Now what do you do? If you're an adult with AS, there can obviously be a lot of landmines, a lot of things to avoid. Here are some things to know ahead of time to make your first date as successful as possible.

The Six Don'ts of Dating

1. Don't monopolize the conversation

Try to think in sentences, not paragraphs. Try not to go on and on about your special interests. Don't start giving the history of all the battles in World War II if you start to feel uncomfortable, or talk about the care and feeding of hedge hogs because you can't think of anything else to say. Try to think of more socially acceptable topics—the weather, current events, the restaurant you're in, etc.

Ask your partner about his or her life. What is she interested in? What are her hobbies? What does she like to do in her free time? Where does she work? Try to think of follow-up questions. For example, if she says she likes to hike, ask her where she likes to hike. If you are familiar with any of the places she mentions, add an opinion or comment: "Oh, I really like Huntington Gorge too. The stream that runs through it is so pretty." This will show you're interested.

Try to stop after a few sentences, though, so the conversation flows more easily. If she likes to listen to the Beatles, ask her what her favorite songs are. Try to have a follow-up question to everything she says—even if you don't know much about the topic. This will help keep the conversation going.

2. Don't focus only on *your* interests

Show you are interested in what *she* has to say. Again, acknowledging what the other person says, asking questions, or just nodding your head is a good way to show you are interested and care about what the other person is saying.

3. Don't tell your life story

This is not the time to be talking about how you didn't make the Little League team at age 10, or got dumped by a girl you really liked in college and you've never quite gotten over it...or the really ugly looking boil on your left foot. Try to keep overtly personal comments to a minimum until you know the person better. Too much information right away can scare a person away.

If the other person starts volunteering more personal stuff, and you seem to hit it off well, then you can follow her lead, but as hard as it is for Aspies, try to stay somewhat superficial at first. You are "testing the waters," so to speak—getting a feel for each other.

4. Don't be a slob

Shower, comb your hair, dress properly. Make sure you have clean clothes that match, and that you've showered. Don't do things like pick your nose or other private behaviors while on the date.

5. Don't go too fast, or be too blunt

You have to take your time. Don't ask her to have sex with you or make references to this on the first date Don't make any crude references to sexual activity. Most Aspies don't like small talk, but most people rely on it as a way to get to know what people are like. You can go into detail more in later dates but try to keep replies short the first time.

6. Don't stress out

Take a deep breath and try to relax. Be yourself, if at all possible—while trying to still follow the advice above as much as you can. Worrying too much won't help.

A Note on Sexual Relations

A person's sex life is obviously a very personal thing. Some people with AS have trouble knowing where their boundaries are, however, and this can be a problem in relationships. Make sure you know now what you are comfortable doing and not comfortable doing in a sexual relationship. Give some thought to your boundaries, and don't compromise them. Set limits. Make sure there is clear communication on the part of both people on what activities you both like, and what you don't like. Make sure to say no if the other person wants to do something you don't like. It is okay to say no. It does not make you a bad person or partner if you say no. You deserve to have your needs respected. If you ever feel unsafe or threatened, be sure to tell someone and get help.

Domestic abuse can sometimes be a problem with Aspies who don't understand that they are being abused. They think it is "just what relationships are supposed to be like." Don't let the other person control what you think, say, do, or whom you see or where you go. If he or she does, it is abuse, even if the person never hits you. Be aware of the different kinds of abuse so you know if you are ever in an abusive relationship, and get help if you find yourself in one.

Final Words

It takes two people to make a relationship work. Adults with Asperger's are more likely to have trouble with relationships due to problems reading social cues, sharing emotions, and communicating effectively. With time and effort, there are ways to work around these blind spots. People in relationships with those with AS may find these behaviors to be frustrating and even insulting, but with time and patience can learn how to understand the AS person and better accommodate their needs. Both people's needs are equally important, and neither should be blamed more than the other for any problems that arise in the relationship. Love may seem like an elusive thing for someone with Asperger's, but it is out there and you can find it. Others have done so successfully. And you can too, in time.

Paul's Story

I was a C and D student all through school. I repeated second and sixth grades finally graduating at 20 and going on to a community college for 3 semesters before working full time.

I grew up enjoying music from folk rock, and from 5 years old, I loved the music of the Beatles to the point I dreamed of being in a rock band and started playing drums. In second grade my teacher told my parents I couldn't play the drums. My parents then bought me an acoustic guitar. I of course wanted an electric but for one year I carried it around as a prop holding it left handed because I idealized Paul McCartney until my father decided it was time for me to take lessons. Through the 70's I built up a repertoire of songs from popular singers of the 70's (James Taylor, John Denver and many others) and played in many talent shows and even played for tips in a bar when I was 16.

I worked in a retail job for almost 30 years while performing for children on dialysis and other gigs for free. After my employment was terminated I started playing and singing at a coffee house and later retirement homes for money.

I went through Vocational rehab while applying for jobs. I was diagnosed with Aspergers through V. R. after I turned 50 and was told one of the jobs I was interviewed for, and was turned down for, was related to A.S. because of the test they gave my answers where questionable.

I am currently employed, as of November, at a shipping warehouse and still doing retirement Gigs. My struggles through school were my failures. My job performance was a challenge. My talents on the guitar became my success.

My new job is going well and I still have the enjoyment of entertaining the old folks. Thank you for reading this.

Sincerely Paul K. W.

***

3. Loving Someone With Aspergers

Problems connecting with others in social situations are a well known attribute for those with Asperger's syndrome—let's face it, when was the last time your spouse or boyfriend looked forward going to a party with lots of people? What many people do not know is that individuals with Asperger's often have difficulty connecting with loved ones as well.

Spouses or others in relationships with Aspies often bear the brunt of the loneliness and isolation that comes with a partner with Aspergers. It is a challenge, but with a little effort and creativity, excitement and fun can be brought into an otherwise one-sided relationship.

Paula's Story

I've been married almost 35 years to my husband who was just diagnosed with AS at the age of 60 years old. I was told he had schizoid personality since he was in his thirties by two different health care providers—a psychiatrist and a psychologist.

Until now I've been in therapy, on and off since before we got married, over our relationship. It was not very easy at times. We did almost break up many times but that just

63

never happened. We've been in therapy together and separated over the years. I would say now it is the easiest. Our two wonderful children are happily married. I do remember my son once saying to me that I act like we're a normal family. I'm almost scared to speak openly about their father's diagnosis because even though we already have one fabulous grandchild I don't want to scare them that maybe they could have a child was autism.

I would say I had to do most of the raising of my children to show them what I wanted for them. My husband threw himself into work. He said just lately that I'm glad I did so I wasn't home much. I do feel sorry for my husband that he didn't get any help that he might have used to understand his behavior more. He did tell me to tell my brother that he's sorry he wasn't more friendly with him because he now knows why he couldn't be. The last thing I would like to say is that I'm sorry my mother-in-law died before ever knowing what her son must of gone through to get by to this point. He does understand his behavior now. It still is hard for me when we have somewhere to go and he gets in a bad mood because he really doesn't want to go. He's so much more comfortable in his own house.

Paula

***

Rekindling Your Relationship

It seems simple but the first thing to do to rekindle the spark in any relationship is to go on weekly dates. Sure the standard movie and dinner is fine, but to really bring it up a notch it is a good idea to go on more adventurous dates. If you are thinking that spontaneity and Asperger's mix together as well as oil and vinegar, you are not alone. Your loved one with Asperger's thrives on routine and ritual, which can often become extremely boring for you. A friend of mine Jo, who is married to a man with Asperger's, expressed how her romantic life had become like Groundhog Day.

"I love my husband Jeff; he is a wonderful man who happens to have Asperger's. When we first started dating he would often think of new things to do and fun places to go, but once we got married all that stopped. Now it is the same thing every time we go out. We go to his favorite pizza parlor, split a pepperoni pizza with extra cheese, and then see a movie. Even though we go to a different movie every so often, the routine date gets stagnant after the 50th time of doing the same old thing. The worst part is the same routine in lovemaking as well. It is always the same thing every time. While vanilla is nice, I would like a different flavor once in a while.

When I mention to him that I would like to venture out and try new things, he grumbles and shoots down every idea I throw out. The zoo is too dirty, the beach too cold, the new French place too expensive. He will make any excuse to keep his safe (and boring in my opinion) routine."

Bring Up the Idea Well in Advance

While many individuals with Asperger's thrive on keeping a set routine in their day-to-day life, as Jo expressed it can be very frustrating for those without Asperger's to keep doing the same thing over and over. The key to persuading your partner to try something new is to mention it well ahead of time. Let's say Jo wanted to try that new French restaurant. She should casually mention that she read a rave review in the paper, with no comments on how she wants to go there, just mention the restaurant. The next day she should say how she has really been in the mood for French food lately. The following day ask if this weekend they would try the new place. Finally Jo should go ahead and make reservations and tell Jeff that day they are going to dinner at the new place at x time. While Jeff will most likely protest, he will not be as resistant to try new things since Jo has given him plenty of time to think about—and be exposed to—the idea of the new restaurant.

Exciting Dates

Here are a few ideas for some new and exciting dates. Remember to avoid extremely loud and crowded places, since crowds and loud noise easily agitate individuals with Asperger's. A dance club or concert would not be the best idea for a date. Adding excitement to your date does not have to be an expensive endeavor. You can get creative in planning an exciting date without spending too much money. With a little bit (well maybe a lot) of patience you can coax your spouse to venture out and try new things to make your date night exciting.

Upcoming Local Events

One creative option for a date is to look online or in a newspaper for upcoming local events. There are many things going on in your town or the nearby cities that are fun, novel and often reasonably priced. Look for certain harvest festivals in the fall. Go to a summer fair and ride the Ferris wheel and eat cotton candy. During the holiday season there are tons of fairs, festivals and other fun activities that would make a great idea for a date. Ask your local library or community center for upcoming events.

There is bound to be something to do that is new and will make for an exciting date. Just make sure to plan to go in off times to avoid the crowds.

Play Tourist for a Day

Play tourist for a day and pretend you are a new visitor to your city. Go see all of the interesting spots that you always drive by but never explore.

Go on a Double Date

Ask different friends for ideas of things that they have done on memorable dates. Going on a double date can add a different vibe to a date. Make sure that you are both comfortable with the other couple, as it may be difficult to really relax for individuals with Asperger's when other people are around and they are expected to interact socially.

Having another couple around can add excitement and help to learn about new ideas for dates that the couple has already experienced.

Go on an Old Fashioned Picnic

Certain romantic ideas never go out of style. Pack a basket with different cheeses, grapes and some champagne and go to the park for an old fashioned picnic.

Other Ideas

Take a romantic stroll on the beach or at a nearby lake and watch the birds. A humanitarian based date can add novelty while giving back to the community. Take your date and give out sandwiches to homeless people. Go to a new park and plant a tree. Volunteer to take your neighbor's dog for a walk. Giving back to the community will give you and your date a good feeling, and create a fun, new memory.

More Fun Ideas

Here are other fun ideas for a date; go ice skating, go to a comedy show, go to an aquarium, go parasailing, go skydiving, go camping, go cart racing, go swimming in a nearby pool, lake or ocean. The possibilities are endless. All it takes is a little creativity, a little coaxing and preparation your next date the most exciting one yet.

Avoiding the Stumbling Blocks

Here are a few stumbling blocks in relationships that are typical of individuals with Asperger's and how to overcome them.

Communication Challenges

The first main issue lies in communication. Often the communication between any couple can become stagnant at times. When an individual has Asperger's, keeping up communication is often a one-way event. Of course it is frustrating to try and bend over backward to communicate effectively, but bringing back communication is the #1 thing you can do to strengthen and bring new life into your relationship. Just sitting down for 5 minutes each day and discussing how things are going can really begin to open up the lines of communication between two individuals. Often when a person with Asperger's comes home from work they are done talking to others and just want to be left alone. Unfortunately for their partner, this habit can create a large rift in a relationship and, overtime, can destroy even the most loving relationship. Make a point to have "we" time. Set aside time during dinner, turn off the TV and really focus on each other. If there is resistance, just try baby steps. Talk for 5 minutes (you can even set a timer) and then watch TV like usual.

Learn to Share His Interests

Loved ones often express that they feel disconnected from their Asperger's partner. Often a person with Asperger's will be fully engrossed in their own hobbies, and shut out all other forms of stimulation. This can be very isolating for a loved one, and often creates feelings of resentment and frustration for both members of a relationship. One thing that can be done to bridge this disconnectedness is to get involved in your partners hobbies. Take a real interest in things that they find exciting. One couple I know said as soon as they started to enjoy similar things, they felt closer and their relationship grew stronger.

"Mark was obsessed, and I mean obsessed with old train stations. He spent hours researching them on the Internet and fantasized about visiting a particular train station in Florida. Well, after night after night of feeling ignored I decided if you can't beat them, join' em. I started looking online at the train station Mark was so fixated on and secretly booked a trip there for the following weekend. I will never forget the look on his face when I told him where we were going. He was so excited. I actually ended up enjoying our trip as well. The whole car ride back we talked about the train station, and I could actually understand and appreciate his passion. We still talk about how wonderful that trip was, and 15 years later we are still deeply in love."

Making a relationship work requires time, effort and a lot of patience. Many people go from relationship to relationship and never can quite figure out how to make a relationship last. Keeping the romance alive in any relationship can be difficult due to the monotony and demands of daily life. Add the stress of having a loved one with Asperger's and maintaining a relationship can seem downright impossible at times. Taking care of the chores, entertaining the kids and focusing on a career can all take precedence over romance in a marriage. A romantic marriage does not mean spending a lot of money on fancy dinners, buying your spouse luxurious presents or writing sappy love letters to one another. Modern day romance can be easily maintained in a marriage with a little effort, patience and communication.

Keeping the Spark Alive

Defining what romance means for a couple is integral in keeping both members of a marriage happy and fulfilled. Just because the media defines romance as a candlelight dinner at a swanky restaurant does not mean that is what is romantic for you as a couple. Perhaps you prefer tulips to red roses or sushi to chocolate covered strawberries. It is important to communicate your likes and dislikes to your spouse so that they can get a better feel for what you see as romantic.

Many spouses (usually of the male variety, sorry guys!) are unsure of how to romance their spouse. They will relay on traditional, well-known methods of romance such as red roses, chocolate and candles because they are known to work and are a safe choice. If you are not into these traditional methods of romance, let your spouse know. Of course many individuals with Asperger's do not always get subtle social cues, so you need to directly tell your loved one what you need to keep the romance alive.

Ideas for Keeping the Romance in Your Relationship

1. Make a list of things you love (roses, chocolate, when your loved one does the dishes). Print it out. Leave it on your loved one's side of the bed.

2. Tell your loved one specifically what you need. Spell it out. Tell them exactly what you desire. Don't be shy.

3. If you want to begin to do more romantic things for your partner, the same rule applies. Listen to your partner. Observe what he or she really enjoys. Notice what colors/flowers/scents your loved ones attracted to. Notice what sort of foods they enjoy. Romance is all about taking the time to cater to your loved one's likes, and giving them the attention they deserve. It is cliché but when you give love you get love back.

4. Another fun idea is to make coupon booklets for one another. This booklet should include "coupons" or certificates for certain things that you know your partner would love. If your spouse loves backrubs and hates to do the dishes, fill the booklet with free 10-minute backrub certificates and a Get Out of Washing Dishes Certificate. It is a fun and free way to tell your spouse you care about them. If your loved one needs help making you coupons use this as a perfect opportunity to tell them exactly what you like. Don't forget to actually use the certificates on one another.

5. Take out a wedding album or look at some old photos of when you two first met. Talk about your early dates and re-live happy memories.

Here a friend Gina describes how her loved one really made an impact on her.

"One year my boyfriend surprised me with a dozen hot pink roses for my birthday. I was blown away not because he gave me roses, but because he had remembered how beautiful I thought pink roses were. I had mentioned, oh about 50 times how pretty pink roses were and how nice it was to get roses etc, basically spelling it out for him that guess what—I LOVE PINK ROSES! In actuality I dislike red roses, and would have been a tad disappointed if given red roses instead. Because my boyfriend was so attentive and remembered what I really liked (because I told him over and over what I liked an did not expect him to read my mind), he made that birthday the most special and romantic birthday I ever had. The best part was at our wedding a few years later, my bridal bouquet was made up of, and you guessed it, pink roses."

Simple Ideas to Spice Up Your Relationship

There are many ways to spice up a marriage without sacrificing too much time or money. Many people rely on fancy second honeymoons and extravagant dinners to rekindle the romance in their relationship. There are many fun and simple ways to increase the love and intimacy between yourself and your partner without breaking the bank.

Date Night

One idea is to make every X day (Wednesday for example), date night. This does not mean that you have to actually go out on a date, but if you have the financial means and a good babysitter for those with children, go for it. Date night should be simple and fun, but the point is to focus on each other. Turn off the T.V. and eat dinner at the kitchen table. Add some nice candles and your favorite music. If you have children put them to bed or distract them with their favorite movie to give you and your spouse much needed alone time. Tell your spouse how beautiful you think they are, hold their hand, rub their knee, you get the point. The action of labeling one night during the week as 'date night' will help to put the focus on your relationship, and remind you that all relationships need tending to. Your loved one with Asperger's will also especially appreciate the routine of making one night a week date night, as this will become a predictable (fun) thing for the both of you and they will enjoy the conventionality of date night. Date night is a great idea if your loved one has Asperger's. Making date night a routine fits into the mindset of an Aspie. The repetitive nature of making Wednesday date night may work very well and bring back a romantic spark for you both.

Making Romance a Priority

The demands of life often get in the way of keeping romance in a relationship. Careers, children, and housework often take priority over your partner. Many couples begin to take one another for granted and stop working on their relationship. They become roommates and completely lose the romantic element of their relationship. Carve out time every week to do one romantic thing for your partner. Gradually increase that to two things per week. Many partners like spontaneity. A common complaint of partners with Aspie lovers is that they are not spontaneous enough. But you have to be realistic about the level of spontaneity you can expect. Schedule these romantic gestures into your planner. Ask your Aspie partner to do the same. If he or she forgets, a little reminder may be needed. It is better to give a little nudge or hint and have the romance build then to have no romantic interludes and end up resentful. These gestures do not have to take a lot of time or effort. They can be as easy as holding hands, or picking up your loved one's favorite take out after they have had a hard day at the office. Slowly incorporating the romance back into a relationship will take time, but gradually things will become second nature and you will not have to work so hard to be romantic.

Keeping a Marriage Happy

Couples often search for marriage advice and tips to ensure a long and healthy union. The divorce rate in this country is over 50% (while statistics are hard to come by for marriages with one Asperger's partner, the divorce rate is reputed to be over 80%) and with the extra stressors of having a spouse with Asperger's, maintaining a happy and healthy marriage can often seem like an impossible task. There is not a particular formula that will create a happy marriage, but here are a few tips to help increase the joy and satisfaction within a marriage.

Don't Forget to Focus on Yourself

The most important tip in a successful marriage is to like who you are as a person. It is cliché but true that you really cannot love another until you truly love yourself. It is also significant to share your particular interests with your spouse and pursuing interests separate from your spouse. If you begin to see yourself only as part of a couple, it is likely you will lose your identity as a person. Fill your own emotional needs; if you do not rely on another person to fill your needs, you will see your marriage more as a partnership. This is very helpful in a marriage where one spouse will often focus intently on his own interests, as those with Asperger's do. Try to let your spouse have space, and see it as an opportunity to pursue your particular interests. Be careful, as always doing separate things can create a rift in a relationship—just try to balance 'we' time and 'me' time.

Be Kind

It sounds simple, but being nice to your spouse is an often forgotten marriage tip. Many treat their spouse differently than their friends, and can often be harsh and sometimes downright mean to their spouse. It is tempting to take life's frustrations out on your spouse—particularly when they are acting quirky as those with Asperger's often do. A good tip is to "bite your tongue" before saying something could be insulting or negative to your spouse. Of course if there is an issue that needs to be discussed and it will involve some negative comments, communication should not be stopped. Just remember that you should talk to your spouse in the same respectful tone you would a stranger or friend—and remind yourself that they struggle with a disorder that makes communication more difficult for them.

Couples within the perfect of marriages will inevitably have disagreements. The tip is to "fight fair" and keep the disagreement on topic without bringing up unrelated issues from the past. Focus on what needs to be resolved and fight so both you, and your spouse, will be satisfied with the outcome, not just to 'win' the argument.

Share Positive Ideas and Ideals

Another tip for a successful marriage is to share positive ideas, experiences and ideals with one another. Share with your spouse a happy thing that happened to you during your workday. Make a list of things that make you both happy and vow to do them more often. Perform random act of kindness not only for a stranger, but also for each other. Buy your spouse his or her favorite flower just because. Compliment and support your spouse. If they have had a bad day listen to them. If they have had a good day rejoice with them. Be their biggest fan. Once you begin to make these small changes, you will begin to see changes in the way your spouse reacts to you and will eventually begin to see improvements within your marriage.

Marriage is Not Always 50/50

One great piece of marriage advice is to recognize that marriage is not always 50/50. Some days you may have to give 90% and your spouse will give 10%. Other days you may give 25% and your husband will have to put in the 75%. The tip to a successful marriage is all about give and take, some days you will have to give more than take. If you begin to feel that you are giving more than taking, communicate with your spouse. If you are taking more than giving, take a step back and look at other resources you can use for support. Many disagreements and disillusions within a marriage boil down to miscommunication. Do not be afraid to talk to one another, just do so in a loving and respectful way.

Communication = Successful Marriage

Marriage often begins filled with hope, joy and happiness, but over time a couple can grow apart and eventually end their union. Being married to an individual with Asperger's can be particularly challenging. People are constantly looking for advice and secrets to create and maintain a healthy and happy marriage. The most important thing in a marriage does not revolve around sex, money, looks or children. The number one factor in determining if a marriage will survive is communication.

Communication is essential to success in all areas of life. To be successful in a career you need to communicate with your coworkers. To be a successful parent, you need to communicate with your children. There is no difference with your spouse than with any other area in your life. Communication is essential for success in a marriage. Individuals with Asperger's often fail in successful communication skills.

Traci's Story

Well, I do not have AS, but there is a strong possibility that my husband might. My hubby was always a "loner" as a child and the strong silent type as an adult. He is coming up on his 33rd birthday. We have been married for 5 years, together for 7 years, and are on the verge of a divorce at this time.

76

Mid-2009, he began to have some unusual behaviors, and simply isolated himself from me and our life together. We began marital counseling shortly after the behaviors surfaced, which is when the potential for AS was identified by our therapist, who seems to be a very skilled clinician. Along with AS, he seemed to be struggling with anxiety and I believe was experiencing panic attacks. He was prescribed Xanax for the anxiety and has found some relief. He has a lifelong history of insomnia and for the first time ever, is sleeping well with this medication. He relayed to me that he must have had anxiety his entire life, but never knew what the feeling actually was.

He had stopped attending marital counseling a while ago, but is just now starting to again participate in sessions. His ability to actively participate seems to be very hindered, having difficulty expressing himself and getting easily flustered when discussing feelings/emotions. He has declined individual therapy and insists on taking his anxiety medication only at this time. His primary care physician wishes to have neuro-psych testing performed, but he will not likely agree. He seems very fearful of labels and diagnosis. I am a trained social worker myself, so the process is understandable for me, which I feel makes him even more distrustful of me, having accused myself and our marital therapist of "ganging up on him". I love him dearly and desperately want our marriage to work, but he won't allow me to help him.

Traci

***

Communicating With Your Asperger's Spouse

One hallmark feature of Asperger's is difficulty communicating in social situations and in relationships. Being married to someone with Asperger's does not mean your marriage is doomed, but it does mean that you will have to work hard at opening up the lines of communication and finding ways to maintain that communication over time. Your marriage will often feel lopsided and you may feel that you are putting in all of the effort while your spouse is just going through the motions. This may in fact be true, and is a challenging aspect of living with an individual with Asperger's. The best thing to do is to remind yourself that your spouse is a different person from you and has their own way of doing things. Just because you feel you are putting in more effort to the relationship does not mean that your spouse does not care and love you just the same.

Couples often fall into routines in becoming comfortable with one another. They rely on previous knowledge about their spouse and figure that they know one another so well that the other has to know what they are thinking at all times. Humans are complex and intricate beings, we are not robots who are programmed once and will never change. People do change, their likes and dislikes shift over time, their priorities change as they get older, and their attitudes change. It is doing your spouse a disservice to assume that they are the exact same person as they day you were married. It is also unfair to assume your spouse will be able to unconsciously know about your changing views. Many individuals with Asperger's will often maintain the very similar likes and dislikes over time, and may assume you do the same. This is why it is so important to communicate to them what you need and desire, as well as inquire what their shifting needs are as well.

How to Communicate Efficiently

Communication in a marriage does not mean expressing every single view, belief or opinion to your spouse. Some times it is better to keep your opinions to yourself (like when you dislike the outfit your spouse is wearing). Main core beliefs and feelings should always be expressed, regardless of the repercussions. Many feel afraid to be honest with their spouse because they do not want to create conflict. Holding back feelings and opinions will gradually build over time and lead to an eventual explosion of aggression against your spouse. This is commonly known as passive-aggressive behavior. A person will often passively hold back feelings or opinions for fear of creating conflict, and will eventually explode and do something aggressive to their spouse, such as 'forget' about that special dinner you two had planned for weeks.

In the moment, speaking one's mind may be intimidating and even uncomfortable, but communicating in the moment is much more effective and healthy that communicating in a passive aggressive manner. It is very common to see passive aggrieve behavior in a marriage where one spouse has Asperger's, due to the inherent lack of communication and feeling as if you are in a one-sided relationship.

Here is an example of a couple whose lack of communication has created a much larger problem in their marriage.

Jack and Cara have been married for 7 years. Jack did not understand why his wife Cara was always nagging him to be more social. "Be more social," she would say. "Come out with my friends. Let's go to the mall". She was always nagging.

Jack has Asperger's and prefers to be alone much of the time. He hates to be in social situations and found it easier to ignore Cara's requests and brush her off time and time again. He did not explain to her that these social situations made him extremely uncomfortable. Cara thought Jack was being rude and inconsiderate of her needs, so she finally started doing things without him. Cara would always feel so embarrassed when her friends would ask why Jack was not with her. Her friends even teased her that she had an 'imaginary husband' because Jack was absent from social gatherings much of the time. This infuriated and frustrated Cara. Eventually they grew apart and Cara started to resent Jack.

Cara and Jack are not alone in their difficulties to establish and maintain effective communication within a marriage. If Jack had been better able to communicate and Cara more willing to work with Jack, perhaps this situation would have a different outcome. Unfortunately shortly after the Holiday season, Cara and Jack separated.

Help With Communication

Of course it can be very difficult when communicating with a spouse because they will often become defensive and fire back at you when communicating. Individuals with Asperger's are often unable and unwilling to fully express their emotions to others, and find it easier to ignore you or turn the tables and begin to criticize you. If you are prepared for this and willing to remain calm and patient, you will be better able to effectively communicate with your spouse.

If you feel like you are unable to communicate with your spouse, perhaps seeking outside help from a therapist would be beneficial. Even one or two sessions with a therapist can provide a much-needed boost to your overall communication and can begin to help repair a distant marriage. A therapist may also be able to make things more comfortable for your spouse to express certain things, as well as help you understand that the way your spouse behaves is due to Asperger's.

Communication is of the utmost importance in keeping a marriage happy and healthy. If you begin to be honest with yourself and with your partner, you both can lead more fulfilling lives and grow closer to one another than you ever thought possible. It will take hard work to get communication back on track and things might become worse between the two of you before they get better. Just remember to have an open mind, and an open heart and embark on the journey to make your marriage the best it can be.

Education and Understanding

Living with a loved one who has Asperger's can pose many challenges. From rigid routines, to closed off emotions, individuals with Asperger's can make it frustrating for all those whom they have an intimate relationship with. Understanding your loved one can work wonders for your relationship. It is important to educate yourself surrounding the typical traits and behaviors of someone with Asperger's. Joining a support group, researching Asperger's on the Internet, and reading books (such as this one) can be good ways to lean more about the general attributes of an individuals living with Asperger's. This knowledge can help you to deal with your partners quirks more effectively as well as have a sense that what your partner is doing is part of his disorder, and nothing against you.

Here is a look at a couple that encountered some difficulties because the typical traits of Asperger's were not understood.

Shelly had been with her boyfriend Hank for a little over 7 months. She could not figure out why he never wanted to meet her friends or family. Every time Shelly invited him to her home for dinner or out for drinks with her friends, he always found an excuse for why he could not make it. One night Shelly burst into tears and asked Hank if he liked her.

Bewildered Hank said he did care about her very much and explained to Shelly that he had Asperger's and that is why he had such a difficult time socially. Shelly read about Asperger's on the Internet that night and was overcome with a sense of relief. She realized his reluctance to meet her friends and family was part of Asperger's and not because he was not serious about her. Five months later on their one-year anniversary, Hank proposed. Had Shelly not been educated about Asperger's she may have misinterpreted Hank's behavior and ended their relationship.

Like anything in life, keeping a relationship healthy and happy takes work. When one person in a relationship has Asperger's, maintaining that relationship can take even more work at times. With effort, creativity and a lot of patience and understanding you can make your relationship the best it can be—and most importantly make sure that the both of you are very happy.

Pam's Story

I do not have Asperger's personally, but my husband and daughter do. Asperger's syndrome was not a formal diagnosis until three years after my husband and I were married, and it would be 18 years and a tumultuous union after that that we discovered he had it. We had no idea that he had this disorder until our daughter, at nine years old, was being tested for it at the suggestion of a complete stranger who happened to observe our daughter on the basketball court.

Not knowing my husband had this condition made for a very difficult and miserable time for me. However, after learning about Asperger's syndrome and now knowing what it is and how to work with it has made my life and our marriage a very workable and enjoyable experience. My husband had been told he had a learning disability when he was a child. But watching him assemble an engine from a box of unmarked, disassembled pieces and seeing it fire up the first time he started it, I was not convinced he had any kind of learning disability. I was angry that he was that smart, but couldn't behave during family gatherings, resisted any kind of social gatherings in an effort for me to socialize, and couldn't help but get angry at children crying or doing anything else that children do. At the same time, he was very sensitive and wanted people to like him and couldn't understand why they didn't.

Nine years into our marriage we had a daughter. She cried intensely for hours at a time as an infant and was terribly difficult to appease. Between her fussiness and his 'quirks', I thought I would go crazy. I contemplated leaving, and actually did leave when our daughter was nearly a year old. We sought marriage counseling, and I could tell that my husband was trying very hard, but couldn't make many lasting changes.

In the meantime our daughter grew older. She was working puzzles at two years old and reading by four years old. She was very smart, also. However, she did not do well with other children at all. She seemed to have a very intense personality and angered easily. One day, I recall, at three or four years old she (in my mind) had earned herself a little spanking. Afterward, she went to her room and literally tore it apart. She raked everything off all the shelves and dresser, took all the bedding off her bed and pulled her mattress off her bed. I had never seen nor heard of any child doing that before. All her check ups at the doctor were within normal ranges and not having any other children, I didn't have anything to compare her to. So I blamed myself for her behavior, thinking I was a sorry excuse for a mother if that was the best I could get out of my child. We tried taking toys away, standing her in the corner, having her write sentences when she got old enough to write, and occasionally spanking her. NOTHING seemed to work except bribery. The child would do anything for a piece of candy.

In the third grade I started to notice a few more things. She was still having temper tantrums when she doesn't get what she wants. When I pick her up from after school care, she would be crying within minutes of getting in the car. At first I was SO sad and disappointed because I hadn't seen her all day and looked forward to getting her at the end of the day, and all she could do was cry hard when she got in the car. I felt like she didn't want to be with me. As the third grade progressed, she started to get the attention of the after school care ladies with some bizarre behaviors with the other children. At this time she is in the middle of her second basketball season. I had noticed that at times she would run with her arms straight down by her sides instead of flexed at the elbows like most people run. She would also get angry if her own team scored because she wasn't the one who had made the shot.

During one basketball game a lady approached me. She introduced herself as a mother of one of my daughter's teammates. She asked me if I had ever heard of Asperger's syndrome. I had not ever heard of it. She then told me she had a teenage daughter with this syndrome and had noticed a few things in Audrey's behavior and performance during the games and practices and asked me to consider the possibility of this for my daughter. Through a fake smile, I thanked her for her information. How dare she point out there was something different about my child?!?! I had known for a very long time that there was something different about her, but as stated earlier, I thought it was my parenting skills. But, out of curiosity I looked up Asperger's syndrome on the internet. I failed to see the correlation between what defines Asperger's syndrome and my daughter's behavior, and she certainly was not autistic!

At the end-of-season party with the basketball team, the mother of the teammate approached me again. The party was held at the YMCA and all the kids were in the pool. My daughter swam by herself until I threw a noodle to her, then the other children began to engage with her. The other mother sat down next to me and this time she told me more about her daughter and less about mine. I was much more open to hearing about her daughter's shortcomings than for her to notice my daughter's.

As it turns out, our daughters had a lot in common. Neither could ride a bicycle for a long time after all the other children were riding. They both insisted on picking the restaurant when we went out to eat. They both had a very easy time with puzzles early in their childhood, and both fared much better when they understood where they were going and what to expect when they got there. The similarities seemed endless. I was forced to take a harder look at the idea that our daughter might have this thing called Asperger's syndrome.

I called the facility recommended by the other mom and scheduled an appointment for our daughter to be tested. After an exhausting day of interview questions for us and interview questions and testing for our daughter, it was confirmed. The doctor stated "Your daughter easily meets the criteria for Asperger's syndrome". It was a bittersweet day that still brings tears to my eyes. It was bitter because no parent wants to know that there is something wrong with their child, but sweet in a) knowing I'm not a bad parent and b) having some answers and possible solutions for what we were seeing with our daughter.

For the fourth grade we enrolled our daughter in a very small private Christian school in the area who is aware of her diagnosis. Although they say they don't have any special needs programs, and are technically not obliged to offer them, the mere environment is a huge plus for our daughter. She is no longer tearful when I pick her up after school, and is in fact quite upbeat at the end of the school day. She happens to be the only 4th grader there, but is in a classroom with two fifth graders and a sixth grader.

As for my husband, the interview questions at the time of our daughter's diagnosis revealed that he too has Asperger's syndrome. Once the criteria was defined and explained to him, he immediately said "That's ME!!" He said he has dealt with this all his life and thought he was crazy. Today he actually owns his own auto repair shop at the edge of a growing town. He manages one employee and is able to enjoy his successes. I am extraordinarily proud of him in light of all he has had to overcome and try to function in a world that is not well-suited for folks like these. The more I learn about Asperger's syndrome the more impressed I am with this gentle giant of a man that I married.

Life in our house is not perfect, and every household has it's own set of challenges. I don't want to leave anyone with the impression that what we experience is any better or worse than what other people must face.

I would like to encourage anyone with Asperger's syndrome to educate themselves and empower themselves with the knowledge of their own difficulties. Our daughter knows she has this, and has been known at times to remind me of it when it seems like I forget. I am forever grateful to the stranger who had the courage to approach me not just once, but twice, to give us a clue! I have called her and her husband to say "thank you" for helping us out.

Pam

***

4. Employment and Adults with Asperger's

Employment. That is the million dollar question, isn't it? We all need money to live on, money to eat with. We need to be able to provide for our every day needs. We need to be able to pay for our homes or rent apartments. We need to go out once in a while and have fun. Unfortunately, though, money usually requires a job. And that is something many adults with Asperger's syndrome (AS) have a lot of problems with.

Some can get disability payments and don't need to work, but others have to. Most want to work just to have a sense of purpose and meaningfulness in their lives. Most people have trouble finding work and keeping work at different times in their lives, but for those with Asperger's the problems can be much more severe. Not understanding social cues, office politics, not coming off well in interviews, having severe sensory issues that interfere with the workplace environment—the list goes on and on. Some adults with Asperger's get lucky and find niches they can fit into, jobs very well suited to their interests. This is the ideal to shoot for. Some need supported employment. There is much to know about the subject of adults and Asperger's and employment, which will be covered in this chapter.

Kathy's Story

I am telling this about my son:

My son is now 31 years old he was born in 1978. No one could ever seem to get a full handle on what was wrong with him. First he was retarded but then he proved that wasn't the problem. He was in some Special Ed classes going through school. He also received speech help and physical therapy classes.

He has had a hard time ever getting a job. People look at him and think that something is wrong with him and he just can't seem to get a job. The government won't help him because they consider him as not wanting to work but that is not true. He has filled out paper work for SSDI but they won't help him with that either. He also had to wear glasses since he was a baby and had hearing problems that added to the problem. Kids made fun of him all the time so he hated to go to school. He went to Job Corps when he was around 21 and he did receive a diploma in Computers but when he got back he just couldn't get a job so he isolated himself in his bedroom and otherwise he would be on the computer all the time.

He now lives in government housing. He had a good relationship for a number of years but the girl gave up and left him because he couldn't get anyone to give him a job. Why won't they just give him a chance? So unfair. Like I said they look at him and just think there is something strange about him and don't give him the chance he deserves. Thanks for reading this.

Kathy D.

***

What are some of the difficulties that adults with Asperger's have getting and keeping a job?

To start, we will talk about the problems those with AS have getting and keeping jobs.

Part One: The Interview

One of the biggest, if not the biggest, problems for adults with AS and employment is getting through the initial interview. You can be the brightest, sharpest person out there, you can know the job inside out, but unless you can connect with the person doing the interview socially, and can come across well, you will never get past the front door.

People with AS do not do small talk well. They might answer questions in a far too explicit manner or say nothing at all; give too much detail about their faults when it is not needed; not look people in the eye and seem excessively nervous and fidgety, which is a sign to most interviewers that they are not prepared or not right for the job—when, in fact, they are like that all the time.

People with AS can be trained in how to get through an interview, how to look people in the eye, how to answer questions the right way. But they are often going to have an air of anxiety pervading them that they can't rid of no matter how much they try, and the interviewers pick up on this and often see them negatively for it. Not all, but a lot of them. Practicing mock interviews with a coach or friend will help a lot. Practicing eye contact, and role playing questions and answers will help give the person with AS a sense of what they should and shouldn't do in an interview, and the kind of questions that will be asked. There are job coaches that are skilled in this, or even friends or family members can help.

Also, the adult with AS will likely need guidance in selecting proper attire for the interview. Does it require a suit, or just a polo shirt? What kind of pants go best with the shirt? Tie or no tie? The way a person presents themselves is very important in an interview; but presentation, and being aware of how they come across, is something that is very hard for most adults with AS.

Ten Job Interview Tips

These are some ways the adult with Asperger's can improve their performance on a job interview.

1. Don't badmouth your past boss

Remember not to talk negatively about your previous job or employer. This only reflects negatively on you and your character. The employer will wonder if you make it a habit to speak negatively of all those you come in contact with. This is not good for workplace morale.

2. Make sure you understand any questions before you answer

If you don't take the time to understand and clarify the question, your answer may make no sense and you may have missed an important chance to show off your strengths. Take a minute or two to compose a thoughtful answer.

3. Try not to appear too desperate

If you seem desperate, it is a turn off. Employers want to hear what your skills are and why you would be a good fit for the organization, not your life story and how you need the job to feed your two kids and ten guinea pigs at home.

4. Don't slouch.

Try to be aware of your body posture and not slouch. Sit up straight as much as you can.

5. Watch your language

It goes without saying you should not curse or use any colorful language. The workplace is not the right place for that.

6. Don't pick your nose

Don't pick your nose or display any other unusual hygiene. This may be obvious but some adults with Asperger's need a little reminder to bring a tissue and comb and to take care of personal issues before the interview starts.

7. Don't complain about anything

If you had to drive around for twenty minutes to find a parking spot, or you think the coffee they served you is too cold, it's probably not the right time to talk about it.

8. Try not to space out or lose attention

If you're thinking about what you're having for dinner that night, the interviewer will probably know.

9. Talk about the job, not your life

Don't give your life story or talk about any problems you are having in your personal life. Stick to talking about the job and relevant, job related experiences you have had.

10. Maintain eye contact

This may be a hard one, especially for those with Asperger's. If you find it really tough to look a person in the eye, then try this trick—focus on the end of the person's nose. Most people cannot tell the difference.

If you follow all these tips, you will have a much better chance of making a good impression on the person who is interviewing you. No one can be perfect, and don't beat yourself up too much if you miss one or two, but do try your best to follow them.

The adult with AS would do well to learn tips to improve their performance on the job interview, but employers could also stand to learn a thing or two to help the adult with AS.

There are many things that a potential employer can do to make the interview process go more smoothly if they are willing.

AutismAtWork.org offers some tips about what someone interviewing an applicant with AS should know and do to try to help the applicant perform better at the interview. The following tips are adapted from the information on their website. If you feel comfortable doing so, or are working with an agency that helps people with disabilities get jobs and they can do so, you might give prospective employers these tips ahead of time.

1. Let the applicant know as much as possible ahead of time

Try to let the person know what will happen ahead of time. Tell them what kind of questions you will ask, and provide a few examples. Tell them how long the interview will run. Tell them what you will do after the interview, for example, call them to let them know your decision, and about the interview process. You might even want to give them a list of questions ahead of time so they will be more able to articulate their answers.

2. Be precise with your language

People with AS need very to the point, explicit language in order to understand what is being asked of them. Speak directly, and if you want to know something, ask. People with AS cannot read between the lines and you need to be very upfront about what you want to know. Small talk is often confusing to those with AS. General questions like "What are you good at?" might be confusing to those with AS; they know there are many things they are good at, but don't know which one you want to hear about. Ask about specific job related skills that you want to know about.

3. Body language

The employer should be aware that people with AS come across very differently when it comes to body language. An adult with AS may sit further away from you or not orient his body in the typical way often expected; it just does not occur to him to do otherwise, or else sitting too close is uncomfortable. Eye contact is a big issue for people with AS. When people with AS try to look into the eyes of another person, often they experience a burning, uncomfortable sensation similar to if you looked into a very bright light. Because of this, they tend to avoid it or not be able to sustain it for very long. This is often seen as being indicative of a bad character or being suspicious in some way; oftentimes applicants are denied on the spot because of this. It is important to remember that the person is still listening to you and taking in everything you have to say; it is

94

just hard to maintain eye contact for that long. They are not trying to be rude. Finally, some people feel that adults with AS will often seem aloof and standoffish, but this is a misconception as well.

4. Amount of information given

People with AS often have trouble gauging how much information to give in response to any particular question. They might go on and on in response to something simple, or only give a few words in response to something that was intended to be a complex question. Feel free to ask for more information if you need it, and also feel free to stop the applicant if he is giving too much information, by thanking them for the answer and telling them you would like to move on to another question.

If you follow all these tips, you will get much more honest, straightforward answers out of the applicant with Asperger's, and get a much more accurate idea of what he can and cannot do. He or she will also appreciate you taking the time to make these adjustments very much, for it enables the person with AS to perform at a level that they otherwise might not be able to achieve.

Part Two: Other Workplace Issues

The difficulties of office politics

As discussed earlier, people with AS do not do well reading hidden messages or understanding subtle social rules of a workplace. They might find themselves in some kind of pickle or social misunderstanding and have no idea how they got there. They might not do enough "schmoozing," or going to company Christmas parties and such, and be seen unfavorably for that, no matter how good their work is.

They may not understand subtle social cues and signals; they won't understand if they are talking too much and a co-worker needs to leave, or that if there is a bowl of candies in the kitchen for people to share, that you should just take one at a time.

They may think people are sincere when they're not, and will take people at face value. Adults with AS have trouble reading between the lines and engaging in small talk. But most typical adults don't like to get too explicit in their communication—they will often try to "sugar coat" or obscure things they want to say. This is just easier for them. They think it is a kinder way to communicate. But they do not understand that the adult with Asperger's may have no idea what they are talking about. Often trying to be more explicit will make them uncomfortable, as they are not used to communicating that way.

Finding Something That Suits the Interests of the Person with Asperger's

If the work is something the person with AS is not interested in, it will be hard for them to be motivated enough to focus on it. This is true for all people, of course, but can be particularly true for those with AS. On the flip side, if it is something they have an interest in, they will be extremely dedicated and loyal, and most likely far more productive than their fellow employees—they actually want to be there and enjoy the work, and they are good at it.

Sensory issues in the Workplace

This can be one of the biggest problems for people with AS in the workplace. Most workplaces are a sensory nightmare. Even typical adults often have trouble focusing and concentrating in office environments the way they are typically set up today.

People talking in the next cubicle, even someone chewing gum or playing with a stapler, or swinging their foot back and forth—everything can be enormously distracting and bothersome to the adult with AS. Food and perfume smells can be hard to deal with. Bright lights, or not enough light, uncomfortable chairs, computer screen glare, even the feel of the telephone as they are holding it—depending on their level of sensory integration difficulty, the workplace can be a very hostile and overwhelming environment indeed for the adult with AS.

And, of course, jobs that demand too much social interaction from an adult with AS can be draining and almost impossible for them to deal with. Some people with AS are good at interacting with the public, most are not. It requires a lot of social savvy and energy to constantly be thinking of what to say, when, how to say it, what words to use, and be aware of how you are coming across. Remembering to communicate in a pleasant tone of voice and manner even if you are angry or frustrated can be hard for all of us, but especially so for the adult with AS.

Emotional regulation

Emotional regulation is one problem that those with AS often have, and they will usually need a lot of downtime and quiet to be able to regulate themselves. Time-outs help them recover from the sensory overload and organize their systems and brains enough to be able to resume the normal office tasks. If you are looking for a job and have AS, try to find one that will let you take these sensory breaks, so to speak, when you need them. Otherwise, the likelihood of becoming extremely overwhelmed, in a short manner of time, is high. Asking for a separate office or trying to work from home as much as possible can solve some of these issues.

Eight Issues to Consider In Selecting a Job

When you are looking for a job that will be friendly to the sensory issues so often found in adults with AS, try to keep these things in mind:

1. Number of employees

How many people work in the organization? How many will you have contact with at any given time, during any given day? How much interaction with people is required in general?

2. Cubicles

Are there cubicles, or will you have an office with a door that you can close? Is there background music playing in the office? Will that bother you? Does anyone have radios playing? What is the general sound proofing like? Are there lots of conversations going on when you walk around—especially if there are cubicles—or does it seem pretty quiet?

3. Breaks

Is there anywhere you can go for a sensory break? A lounge or break room that is separate from the rest of the building? Maybe a bench outside if the weather is good?

4. The boss

Does the supervisor seem understanding and knowledgeable about sensory issues? Does he or she seem like they will be able and willing to accommodate your needs?

5. Lights and odors

Try to notice the lights in the building. Will they bother you? Is there anything you can do to help filter the light if they do? Take notice of if there are any other sensory things likely to bother you; are you too close to the kitchen, where you will smell people's food cooking? Do the perfumes of co-workers get to you? Try to notice these things before you accept a job so you can best gauge if you will be able to handle it and perform well once and if you do get the job.

6. Meetings

Are there a lot of meetings you will be expected to attend? Is there anyone in the organization who you think could help you interpret social situations you may have problems with?

7. Deadlines

Are there strict deadlines or will you be allowed to pretty much go at your own pace? How do you do under pressure?

8. Commuting

How long is the commute from your home? Will you need to take public transportation (and, if so, does it go to your job), or can you drive? Are the logistics of the commute something you feel you can handle?

If you ask yourself all of these questions and any other ones you can come up with, you will be more likely to find a job that will fit your sensory needs. If you are not careful in finding a job that fits your sensory needs, you may find yourself burned out in a very short time. Failures are not fun for anyone and can tend to make one bitter towards working in general, so it is best to choose carefully. Of course, one should keep trying even if a job does not work out, but do choose with care. Some jobs are just better suited for people with AS than others. Examples of such jobs will be discussed later in the chapter.

Farm Boy's Story

I grew up during WWII, long before the original Asperger's syndrome (in German at that time) was translated and noticed by American doctors. I walked to grammar school which had only two rooms, so the grade classes were quite small, and my interactions with others in my age group were limited. I grew up on a family farm, before TV, where children were assigned chores to help the family survive. I milked cows by hand, picked up eggs, and participated in seasonal farm operations. Looking back at it, I don't see how I could have had a better preparation for life with Asperger's at that time.

High school involved a half hour school bus ride, so I did not participate in after school activities. I had signed up for classical studies in preparation for college due to my mother's insistence. But by the end of the first year, I was developing more interests in learning how mechanical and electric appliances worked and how to repair them when they failed. Also courses in electricity and radio were available at the high school, but I could not receive credit for them without changing my group of courses. So I managed to flunk Latin (on purpose), so I could change to the general series of courses.

New products were very difficult to buy, both because of the slow recovery from the depression and rationing due to WWII. When farm equipment failed, I usually volunteered to take it apart and try to repair it, without purchasing new parts. I bought a second hand electric welder and learned how to use it. Radios of that time had five tubes and often failed to operate after only a few years of use. I collected failed units and learned how to repair one by using parts from another, after developing a friendship with the owner of a radio repair shop. At high school, I took interesting classes in typing, electricity and radio, with better grades, even a final average of 100 in radio.

As I approached graduation from high school, the Korean peace action was in progress and the military (army) draft was very active. I learned about a radio and TV repair school that was offering a contest for a two year scholarship, so I signed up. Many of the test questions involved mechanical gear ratios, directions of rotation, use of pulleys and belts which I found easy to solve. I was notified as winner of the full scholarship, so my deferment was extended.

I was able to commute from the farm, except during winter months when I took a part time job working in the school's stock room for night classes. The courses involved solving electrical problems using a slide rule, use of meters and oscilloscopes, practical repair projects on electrical appliances, theory, operation and repairs of radios and black and white TVs. Learning this way from organized courses was far easier and more beneficial than trying to learn things on my own at the farm, and as a result I had the top grade of my class. Before graduation, I visited a navy recruiting office and was assured that my training in electronics would be related to assignments in the navy, so with my father's approval I joined the U.S. Navy.

During my four year Navy enlistment, I was able to take and pass each scheduled advancement test, so I was at pay grade E6, six months before receiving my honorable discharge. I feel this rapid advancement was the result of both special abilities allowed by my Asperger's syndrome and my choice of study courses in mid high school. Even then, I was aware that working with things (electrical equipment) was easier for me than working with people. Equipment follows rules of operation, set up during its design until some failure occurs, and the symptoms of that failure usually lead to its repair back to normal. However people are supposed to follow rules, but each person tends to adjust the rules to their advantage, so the final resulting action cannot be depended on by an observer.

I feel that the decision I made back in high school to flunk Latin was the important turning point that led to my series of successes. It was impossible for me (or anyone) to accurately predict the future, but preparation for possible changes should be considered early in life. Too many people merely continue to live life as it comes, without trying to improve day to day living. There are many things we cannot change, but try to keep aware of opportunities that often occur as challenges you can accept with dignity. While in the Navy, I met many others who were married. Usually their time away from home was a considerable disadvantage which often led to problems or complete separation. I had never even dated, mainly due to my lack of social abilities.

After my time in the Navy, I returned to the farm. My father had died a year before, so I tried to manage and work the farm while commuting for Electrical Engineering courses at college, financed by the GI bill.

I met a young lady in one of my classes and we shared common interests. We married after her graduation from college and before my last year there. After my graduation, I applied for and received a civilian job with the Navy in the field of experimental sea tests, leading to the design of new sonar equipment.

Just before retirement, I had come across literature about Asperger's syndrome and noticed how well the symptoms matched symptoms I had lived with all my life. For me the lack of social abilities seems the most critical. I have learned to suppress feelings of anger or frustration with others who seem so self centered and uncaring of other people. I am frequently bothered by tickling hairs touching my ears or clothing tags that scratch my neck. I detest sports that have become nothing but a relaxed watching of sport for others on TV. But I would never want to be cured of these minor problems if I had to give up the many learning benefits I have enjoyed from Asperger's symptoms.

I have run into a recent problem. When I shared Asperger's information with my wife, she seems to think that once I have identified a symptom, I should be able to eliminate the symptom by entirely ignoring it. I have yet to make her happy that way. For example she does not like my frequent "Stupid light" comment about a traffic light that should be synchronized with nearby others so traffic can continue moving without random, unexpected stops. Too often traffic light installers reduce costs by eliminating features that could have smoothed traffic flow.

Sincerely,

Farm Boy, retired

***

Communication Issues

One issue that many adults with AS run into when they get hired for a new job is frequent miscommunication with their employer and co-workers. People with AS need information to be presented in a very explicit, rather blunt way in order for them to understand it. As mentioned before, they do not read between the lines very easily. Most people do not talk or communicate this way. Employers and co-workers need to be taught to communicate more clearly.

Many adults with AS need information presented to them in a step by step fashion. They will often need to write down the steps to complete a task, and it will require more patience than usual from their supervisor. Some adults with AS are not very confident in their ability to perform tasks on their own. They may need more guidance than the supervisor is able to give. This is where job coaches, provided by agencies who work with people with disabilities, can often be very beneficial.

An adult with AS, given the instruction "Get to work," may look around at them, see everyone else working, and have no idea what they are supposed to be doing. Sometimes, they will be too scared to ask. If they can't advocate for themselves and ask for more help, their job could be at risk. Training for employers on how to best communicate and work with those with AS in the workplace is often needed for an adult with Asperger's to succeed in the workplace.

Adults with AS find it hard to organize and understand information unless presented in a very logical and explicit way. Information and instructions have to be presented very clearly and often written down step by step. No assumptions can be made. An adult with AS will often be overwhelmed with an instruction to "get to work," look around them, see everyone working, and have no idea what they are supposed to be doing (and be too scared to ask), if information has not been presented clearly.

John's Story

Craig, I hope to contribute, but not just at present, as I am driven to distraction by problems.

An Aspie is like a juggler who can keep one ball in the air at a time, but struggles with more than one. Right now I am battling with four or five balls (problems) that just do not seem to get resolved and at times, like today, my mind is on overload and cannot cope—it just goes blank, I forget things, lose things, which are uncharacteristic. Can you recommend anything to help me, please?

John

***

Best Jobs for Those with Asperger's

Now that we have gone over some of the problems that adults with Asperger's often face in gaining and keeping employment, let's look at some of the places in which AS people often excel. Yes, they do exist! There are certain jobs that are just tailor made for the traits of people with Asperger's—and certain jobs, while not perfect, are just a better match for people with AS.

Seven Job Traits of Good Asperger's Jobs

1. Not too much going on at once

Adults with AS are often bad at multi-tasking. Answering the phones, filing papers, doing work at the computer AND greeting people who come into an office, for an example, would have most adults with AS on overload within an hour or less. However, a job that involves only filing, only computer work, or one other solitary task that can be done on the person's own time, in a quiet space, will work much better.

2. Favorable sensory environment

Adults with AS have many sensory issues to contend with in the workplace, as mentioned before. Try to find a workplace without too much noise, with as much privacy as possible, where the adult can control his environment as much as possible. Jobs where you can work from home work well for some people with AS because they can completely control their environment and be able to focus on the work they need to be doing.

3. Fits Your Special Interest

One man with Asperger's said he really enjoyed his job as a clerk in an outdoor gear store, because he got to talk about his special interest all day. If you have an interest in what you are doing, the work will come much easier, and go by faster, and you will be able to cope with the demands of the environment better.

4. Limited Interaction with the Public

Most people with AS find that they get overwhelmed having to deal with social interaction for hours on end. It can be too taxing and take up too much limited energy. Jobs where one can do a task on their own, and go at their own pace, are usually ideal for someone with AS.

5. Jobs with some measure of predictability and routine

Most people with AS do not deal well with surprises. They need to know what is happening at all times. Jobs where a routine is followed, and a schedule is set for each day, work best for the adult with AS. Jobs where your tasks are different each day, you work at different locations each day, or you never know what you will be doing next are very bad for adults with AS.

6. Attention to Detail

Jobs that require attention to detail, patterns or doing the same thing over and over are a good fit for many with AS as they appeal to their natural aptitudes in this area.

7. Working independently

Jobs where you can work on your own instead of part of a team, and go at your own pace, are usually a better fit for those with AS.

Why Adults with Asperger's Make Good Employees

Despite their difficulties in some area, adults with AS often make ideal employees. They are loyal, honest and hard working. They will work to understand how to do a task and they won't stop until it is done right. They don't engage in office politics, which can be a good thing; they will be straightforward with you. They mean what they say. They don't waste time with water cooler chit chat or trying to climb the social ladder. They can often be some of the most productive and hardest workers in an office, once they understand how to do something and have the proper space and accommodations in doing it. Some employers will recognize this and some won't.

Great Aspie Jobs

These are jobs that involve a lot of attention to detail and the ability to work alone. In general, many with AS do well in jobs that involve:

- computer programming
- math
- statistics
- writing
- languages
- research
- working in a library as a reference librarian
- professor at a college
- the arts if they are into this
- engineering

Visual thinkers

More specifically, to break it down even further, visual thinkers might do well in fields like:

- photography
- animal trainer
- commercial art
- small appliance repair

- lab technician
- video game designer
- computer animation
- drafting
- building maintenance
- web page design

Information oriented

Adults with AS who are more into cognitive endeavors, more information oriented, might do well in the following fields:

- library science
- journalism
- accounting
- engineering
- copy editor
- filing jobs
- inventory control
- statistician

If you can't interact with people well or are nonverbal, you might want to consider jobs like:

- re-shelving library books
- janitor jobs
- factory assembly work
- warehouse work
- data entry

- mowing lawns

- restocking shelves

A recent discussion on the Asperger's website WrongPlanet.net had many people weighing in on what jobs worked well for them, and what didn't.

User KittenFluffies said, "My favorite job was a three-month position as a researcher for a professor in the History Department. I made my own schedule, got to read all day, and worked independently in the library (nice and quiet). This job made good use of my visual-spatial & reading skills (I'm a speed-reader). It also helped that it paid quite a good bit. I wish I could do it full-time. This is the job that made me realize I want to be a Research Librarian when I grow up. Heh. Right now I am an office manager/copywriter at a Real Estate firm. It sounds terrifying but the office is small, quiet and I have my own office to myself. However, I would rather not do this all my life as it is not very fulfilling or stimulating."

User Lotuspuppy spoke to what a person does when they can't find a job that is a career, but just need a job that takes place in a sensory environment they can tolerate and provides a paycheck:

"A ton of other Aspies I have met are mail-room sorters. Obviously, that is a bit low on the pay-scale, but I think that any job with sorting is really good for us. Even in my office job, where I deal with people in a semi-unpredictable environment, I still enjoy the stability of entering data into an Excel spreadsheet."

User Lannesman defied the idea that people with AS can't work well the public by talking about his job selling movie theater tickets. He says, "Movie theatre ticket seller. You are in a small box. Mostly alone. You speak to people thru a mic. Bullet proof glass separates you from unclean people. Everything has a place. The show times are absolute. The prices are absolute. The R rating is absolute ("Sorry, you are not of age and have no parent or guardian with you"). No one can reach out and touch you. And if anyone has a problem in the show they are already inside and must take it to the manager."

Finally, user Cage Aquarium suggests being a security guard of some sort, due to the amount of time spent alone and low demands of the job. "If you happen to be an Aspie and did not come equipped with the standard Aspie genius module such as me I have found you can't beat security work. All night I sit at a gate talking to maybe 3 people a night in short one word sentences with zero eye contact because I was taught to watch people's hands when I talk to them on duty. Otherwise my job requires me to sit alone and stay awake occupying my time with whatever I please so long as I keep my eyes on the gate sensors and do a foot patrol every once in awhile. Gives me all kinds of time to write and draw so that is one I'd suggest."

As you can see, there are many different avenues an adult with Asperger's can explore to find a job that fits them, from researcher, to mail clerk to security guard. The key is finding a job that works with your unique strengths and weaknesses, in an environment that you feel comfortable in.

Creating Autistic Friendly Work Environments

People with Asperger's and other autism spectrum disorders often have unique skills and traits that can be of huge benefit to a company, but need a very specific environment to work in to be able to function. One company in Denmark is leading the way in developing a new concept—workplaces made up almost entirely of adults with Asperger's. Such environments can allow employers to create an environment that better suits the needs of this population, while allowing them to produce superior work. There is no supported employment or a workshop; adults work at market rates.

In an article published in the May 31, 2009 Independent UK newspaper, entitled "Better, Faster, and With No Office Politics: The Company with Autistic Specialists," Thorkil Sonne of the company Specialisterne explains why developing an IT (information tech) company of adults with AS was such a good idea: "There are so many different types of phones and services to be tested," Sonne explains. "And the work is very repetitive but requires full attention all the time. Most companies use students or outsource to India or wherever. The first couple of tests they'll do will be fine, but by the sixth, their attention wanes and it will always be the last test that's the most important." Aspergerians, on the other hand, relish the repetition, their focus doesn't waver and their numerical skills are superlative. "My staff are motivated all the time. Our fault rate was 0.5 per cent, compared with five per cent from other testers. That's an improvement by a factor of 10, which is why we can charge market rates. This is not cheap labour and it's not occupational therapy. We simply do a better job."

This venture shows that not only can adults with Asperger's be useful employees, in many cases they can outperform their typical peers, given the right working conditions.

Sonne goes on to explain, "It is a relief to work with colleagues for whom office politics, backbiting and bitchiness are anathema. They are a happy and loyal group, no one ever talks badly about anyone else. It's nice to work with people who are honest, without filters. In fact I am working on a new management technique based on our experience with working conditions that are more open and direct."

With benefits like this, it is no wonder more employers are starting to see why they should hire employees with Asperger's. In fact, such benefits might even be worth putting up with the occasional social gaffe—like the employee in Specialisterne, who, Sonne reports, "had to be told, when we introduced a free fruit basket, that you only take one or two at a time instead of half the basket." Yes, such social gaffes seem well worth it to get a whole new generation of people into the workforce who might not have been able to work otherwise—and who produce such useful results for their employers.

Jobs that Do Not Work for People with AS

Any job that requires too much focus on the short term memory, remembering too many bits of information at once, and multi-tasking will probably not be a good fit. Any job that requires prolonged contact with the public is not often a good fit.

Specifically, things like being a waitress would be difficult because there a lot of different tables to keep track of it at once. A cab dispatcher, or any kind of dispatching job, would be the same. A receptionist job would be difficult when the switchboard got busy. Being a cook, for example a short order cook at a restaurant, would be hard because of the same problem—doing too much at once. Ideally, you want a job where you can do one task at a time.

A Word on Freelance or From Home Jobs

One ideal option—if you can get it—for people with AS are freelance jobs. In other words, work for yourself, and in a lot of cases, work from home. This can range from photography and design, to writing, to something using the telephone, to daycare. If you can create your own business and market it and do it from home, you will have a much better working environment. Some people find that telephone work, as long as it involves only making outgoing calls and not having to deal with a lot of incoming calls at once, works well for them, because often you have a particular script you need to follow and you are not allowed to deviate from it. This repetition works well for some people with AS. Some telephone jobs allow you to work from home with a phone and Internet connection. Also, sometimes you can do data entry jobs from home, if you can get the information you are working with over the phone.

Help in Finding and Keeping Employment

It is great if you can follow a traditional road to employment or even a not-so-traditional one but still work independently. But some people need more help than that. There are several options for adults with AS who want to work but need more help staying on task, learning new tasks, staying directed, or navigating the environment socially.

Job Coach

One such thing is a job coach. A job coach is like a shadow that will help you figure out how to do your job. They will help you interact with your supervisor, talk to them about your disability, and be there to answer any questions that might come up during the day. If you go to the Vocational Rehabilitation, or Voc Rehab, office in your city, they can often set you up with one. Voc Rehab is a great resource for anyone with a disability to get help figuring out how to get a job and to get the necessary help in securing a job. Sometimes Voc Rehab will pay for college for someone who needs more education to get a job. Sometimes they will help with transportation for a job. Sometimes they will pay for necessary equipment or training for you to be able to succeed in a job. There are a lot of different things that Voc Rehab can do to help.

More About Voc Rehab Services

In order to apply for Voc Rehab, you must be a legal US citizen, have a physical, mental or emotional disability that keeps you from finding or keeping a job, and be somehow willing and able to work in some form.

Voc Rehab counselors will talk to you about your disability and how it interferes with your ability to work. They will discuss your education, experience, knowledge, skills, and interests. Your work history and abilities will also be discussed. Any kind of assistive technology you might need will be examined.

The services Voc Rehab may offer are quite varied and depend largely on your personal situation, and also the office you are working with. Medical, psychological and social assessments may be done, to see if you need any help in any of those areas. Medical care to help you be more able to work might be offered. Job training, volunteer experiences, and transportation might be something that will help you. Job coaches that help you on the job are another idea. Usually, there is a waiting list to get Voc Rehab services, so it is best to put your name in as early as possible.

Supported Employment

Some adults with AS want to work but need more help in the workplace. One option to help with this is called a sheltered workshop. These are usually organizations that have jobs that people with disabilities can do that offer a lot of support. One organization defines sheltered workshops this way: "Sheltered workshops are state supported vocational programs designed to provide work for persons with mental retardation/developmental disabilities." (http://www.rcomo.org/whatisasw.htm)

Sheltered workshops can be found in most cities. Ask your local Autism Society of America chapter, or your doctor, for referrals to local places.

A less restrictive form of help with employment is supported employment. The state of New York defines supported employment in the following way: "Supported employment programs provide people with severe mental illness with direct placement in jobs in competitive, real-world settings with accompanying on-site and as-needed support services, which are designed to help individuals perform their job."

The key here is that the adult with AS gets coaching and help directly on the site of the job; their questions are answered, their anxiety soothed; they are able to focus on their job and have the feeling of self-accomplishment and sufficiency that comes with holding down their own job—as well as getting a paycheck from that job.

What if you can't work at all?

For those who are not able to work at all, it is possible to apply for Social Security Disability or Supplemental Social Security Income to be able to pay for some of your living needs.

A Personal Perspective — Issues in the Workplace for Adults with Asperger's

To close this discussion, we will take a detailed look at the experiences of one woman with Asperger's experience in the working world—her challenges, the things that went well and what ultimately ended up working for her. Reprinted with permission.

"What a subject—adults with Asperger's and jobs. As an adult, I have not been able to tolerate much in the way of employment. I do some freelance work but most traditional

116

means of employment are closed to me, due to severe sensory issues, and not being able to understand directions as quickly as I need to, not being able to understand office politics, not being able to handle more than one thing happening at a time, and so on.

I had a few jobs when I was in high school and college, but none lasted long. I didn't seem cut out for work; everything seemed foreign, I just didn't seem to be able to fit in or follow directions very well. Just all sorts of problems. Even in jobs that you think would be better suited for someone with AS. I never went for any retail jobs or any jobs where you had to stand on your feet all day or talk to people or do a lot of things at once; I couldn't even imagine being able to do that. It's not that I'm lazy; I just break down after doing any of that stuff for an hour. Anyone could see that. I wanted to.

But there were two jobs I did have. One was working for a mapping company. They made maps, and used computers to plot data to generate the maps. It was a low key relatively quiet environment; just sit at the computer and plot your data. Thirty hours a week. I lasted the entire summer but it didn't work out well. First, I couldn't understand what I was supposed to be doing, exactly, and would ask the supervisor, but they never seemed to be able to tell me in a way that made sense to me. I thought I was doing okay, and doing it accurately enough, but I could never understand why I was so much slower than all the others. I would get overwhelmed because there was a room with 15 people and they would all be talking at once, and I couldn't get any work done. I didn't even think of asking to be switched into the other, quieter room until halfway through the summer, but even then it was hard. I felt very uncomfortable and ill at ease around the other workers, especially at break times. Everyone else would socialize, and talk to each other, and I would be left standing alone. This was very depressing to me. Even though I did make it through the summer, I wasn't asked back the next summer, and wouldn't have really wanted to go back either.

The second was better in some ways but worse in others. It was working for a market research company. The good was I had a script to use; all I had to do was sit in my chair and make outgoing calls to people. If I got them, I would use the computer prompts to ask them a series of survey questions. Most of the time, people did not answer the phone and you didn't have to ask the questions. When people did answer and agreed to take the survey, I actually enjoyed it. It was a form of social interaction that was regulated by a script and therefore very easy to do; you couldn't mess it up, and it was fun to hear people's responses. The problem was, in a four hour shift I'd be lucky if ten people answered the phone at all and if two people took the survey. Most of the time you listened to a dial tone over and over again. That got boring. It might have worked, except for the sensory issues. It was open seating and very noisy with people making calls and talking all the time. People's perfumes started to bother me. They renovated the office next to us and the fumes from the new carpet started making me sick, so I had to leave.

In college, I had a job being the monitor for the computer lab at my school. That worked out fine; all I had to do was sit at the computer and answer an occasional question. Put more paper in the printer once in a while. I basically got paid for using the computer. The problem is it's hard to find jobs like that in real life outside of a college setting, and my sensory issues are worse than they used to be, so I couldn't do that now. So I do some freelance work from home, which helps a little, and I also get disability. It's hard to find jobs that suit you when the world overwhelms you so much and so easily. I have found working from home to be the best fit. It gives me more flexibility and more comfort, to be able to work from my home and make my own schedule."

Final Words

The subject of employment and jobs for adults with Asperger's can be a complicated one. There are all kinds of factors one needs to consider. Every adult with AS has such varying needs. One person might do okay in a slightly higher paced job with some public interaction, another might hit overload within five minutes. Some need solitary jobs with routine tasks, others need more stimulation. Some need extra support, some are more independent. Each person is unique. When you consider your options for employment, you need to think about your own strengths and weaknesses. Every adult with AS can do something—even if it is only for a couple hours a day, a few times a week. The right job is out there; you just need to keep looking for it. With the tips in this chapter, hopefully you will be well on your way to finding the ideal job for you.

Alistair's Story

I am a Portuguese SW Engineer who received recently an AS diagnosis. Since I was a kid, many people noticed odd things about myself. At two years old, I used to go to a day care center while my father finished his engineering studies in college and those in charge complained to him that I preferred to be alone playing with my toys instead of playing with the other children. And since a young age, I've always had peculiar interests, like knowing the capital cities of all countries in the world, the different specializations doctors can have, deep water fish species, the names of the stars and constellations, human body organ names, just to name a few. But, although Dr. Hans Asperger had already published his works, there was not a big interest in this difference at the time, especially in Portugal. So I was taken to just be shy, a little odd, but a fine child.

When I was researching AS on the internet, I took lots of online tests and questionnaires available online and all of them, no exceptions, pointed to Asperger's Syndrome. Having diagnosed myself, I decided to consult with a Professor at medical university who is the most known Portuguese specialist in this syndrome and he immediately confirmed my diagnosis. I asked him why I can't master the rules for social interaction when I was able to master the rules of (apparently) more difficult subjects and his answer was very simple: There is not an algorithm for the social interaction, no set of rules you can follow.

And it made sense for me, when in social situations, I've always found myself "working", it takes effort. Something that is natural for other people is not for me. For me it is more relaxed to do a long trip driving a car than being with people socially. With a car, there are precise rules for how it works, gears, clutch, brake :)

For me, social interaction is a major challenge. It is something that I have to be conscious of. It simply is not automatic for me. But this is not critical because for me, it is not especially hurtful (as it is for a neurotypical person :-) to be alone

I'll try to describe you my biggest challenge/failure now.

Since I started my professional life, I've been struggling to answer a very painful and disturbing question: Why are my performance and reward (job satisfaction) so far behind my performance and reward during my academic life?

As a student, I've never had major problems. I always had a very good performance. I finished high school as the best student from my high school. When I arrived at university, I continued to have good results. With few exceptions, I enjoyed studying every subject.

I had high hopes for my professional life about to begin. I was expecting to find friendly environments and projects that would absorb me in such a way that I wouldn't think on anything else, as always happened in high school and university. But today, it seems that wasn't to be :-(

120

The professional world seemed to me radically different from the university. Something had to be wrong, because I simply couldn't get the same enjoyment, the same focus of mind from my projects. This would soon translate into a lack of motivation.

During the years I've done a lot of effort to try to understand why I am not so happy and don't get the same job satisfaction as I did in university and why I cannot take my professional projects in an obsessive way as I did in university. I came up with some possible explanations:

Unlike university there is not a clear text with the precise description of what should be done, the messages are usually transmitted orally and the bosses usually lack the patience to explain the details of the things, rather they expect me to figure them out, even when there are ambiguities.

Again, unlike university, the requisites are not frozen, rather they change wildly, sometimes more than once a day, which is something that "kills" the mental plan I devised, forcing me to start all over. This one, in particular, is a source of much stress for me.

Also, I have a very big need for silence, and I've never been able to isolate myself from the outside noise and talks to properly focus on the job at hand. And, at university, I was able to go home and quietly focus and work on a project. At a company, I get minute-by-minute control from bosses. People breathing on my neck is also a big source of stress for me.

When I'm given some job to do, I enjoy doing it in a very careful manner, so the final result can be the best possible. But most of the time, people seem to be in a big hurry, requesting things to be done very quickly and if needed, with a suboptimal solution and without doing the proper rigorous tests. And, after the job is done, it is not uncommon for me to realize that indeed, there was not a real need for such a big hurry. This causes me, at first, lots of stress, and in the end, lots of disappointment.

My lack of so called social skills has been a tremendous handicap for establishing good working relations and properly working as part of a team. There were a couple of exceptions, of course, I had some "buddy" colleagues with whom I was able to work perfectly as a team, but they were the exceptions, not the rule.

A few years ago, I decided to invest in a post graduate Master course (as a worker student) again in software engineering (specialization in computer networks and distributed and parallel computing systems), for the sake of keeping my skills up to date and marketable. This time, also to know other realities, I chose a different university, but also one with a good reputation. Once more, I enjoyed studying and doing my academic projects and I finished with a good score average (17 on 20 maximum). It seemed my skills were still OK, but that simply wouldn't work in the company world.

I did a lot of research on the internet, trying to figure out what could be my problem, I consulted some specialists that prescribed me some drugs and advised me to "practice" my social skills. But nothing worked, no matter how hard I try, I simply couldn't understand what people meant with their body language and voice changes. This was the source of lots of misunderstood and unpleasant situations that have just kept my work motivation low.

All in all, this is the major challenge, and until now, the biggest failure because I have been unable to overcome it, so far. Unless I find a company who can create an Aspie friendly work environment, (or I create one myself, who knows) I don't see how I can overcome. It is not uncommon to find people who managed to succeed just because of their abilities to play the social game, people who are not particularly brilliant, something simply impossible to an Aspie. It is in this sense that the AS has mainly limited my life.

If it is to point out a big success, I would point my academics performance, but I find it sad to realize that (in the Portuguese society at least, no generalizations to the rest of the world) this is not as appreciated as are the social skills.

Well, I like to travel a lot, I know many places, like north of Europe and several American states and I find the people's mentality quite different from the Portuguese. So, I don't want to talk about "world", just about Portuguese society, the one I am inserted and currently live in. I have to say that I am very resentful and haven't made peace with it. As I explained above, people here consider very important the "superficial impressions". And that places me always in a disadvantageous situation. It is very difficult to sell myself.

I'd like to talk a little about relationships. In the beginning it was difficult, because, being an Aspie, I don't master the body language needed to "know girls at pubs". Needless to say that I've never had much success in that aspect.

This challenge was overcome with the event of internet. On the internet, the body language is not used to communicate. It is mainly just verbal/textual language, something that is not a handicap to an Aspie, pretty much the opposite. On the internet it is not hard to show my inner-self to a female, and, latter to show the outside. This is precisely the opposite of what happens in the non-virtual world. First the outside, and later the inside. And, here in Portugal, it doesn't matter how beautiful the inside can be, if the outside looks "awful".

Best,

Alistair, a Portuguese Software Engineer

***

5. Services for Adults with Asperger's

Sometimes adults with Asperger's can look pretty normal on the outside, but it doesn't mean that on the inside, there isn't a fair amount of things that sometimes need attention and help. It is what is called an "invisible disability"—you look normal, but you still have unique challenges and blind spots. This phenomenon is made harder by the fact that people with AS are often so intelligent in many areas. They have book smarts, can tell you a multitude of facts, can very astutely grasp subject areas that might take someone else four years of college to understand. There are some areas in which adults with AS are far ahead of their peers. They can often fix computers without a manual or a second thought, play complex violin pieces or talk about aerodynamics like it's a fairy tale.

But then why can't they tie their shoes, cook a simple meal without burning it, remember to take their medications or go to a grocery store without having a meltdown? Why do the simplest things confound and bewilder them to the point of overload when they are able to do so much else? It's all part of the puzzle of Asperger's. The way the Asperger's brain is wired seems to create a very uneven profile of abilities and disabilities. Adults with AS end up with some very unique needs that often times are not recognized as valid. If you are an adult with AS, what kind of help can you expect? What kinds of services are available? Where do you turn? This chapter will cover some of those questions.

Common Needs

First, let's talk about some of the needs that adults with Asperger's may have.

1. Social

Adults with Asperger's often end up being isolated due to their difficulties with peer relationships. When you are alone all the time, worries seem bigger, obsessions seem stronger, everything seems harder. It is very good for mental health to get out of the house at least once a day and be able to engage in activities that make you feel connected with the world. Otherwise everything can seem to be caving in on you. Adults with AS sometimes need help getting out and accessing the world. Some adults with AS need help going out to take walks, going to a store or coffee shop, shopping, doing errands and that kind of thing.

2. Financial

Some adults with AS cannot work or cannot work enough to meet their financial needs. For these people, disability payments and food stamps are available.

3. Housing

Some adults with AS need housing assistance financially, and this is where things like Section 8, which subsidize housing, come in. Other people need things like supported housing, or group homes, where their needs can be taken care of or helped by staff members.

4. Everyday household tasks

Simple, everyday tasks can often be overwhelming to adults with AS. They may worry excessively over whether they are doing something right, or what order to do it in, or not be able to interrupt their routine long enough to do certain tasks. This can apply to cooking, cleaning, or any manner of tasks.

For example, following recipes might be difficult because of worry about certain steps or perceived dangers: "What if I use too much cinnamon? How do I know how much to use? How do I tell when the chicken is done? Is that safe to eat? How do I get that sticky stuff off of the bowl? How long do I need to clean it for? How much butter should I put in? What should I mix in first?" Things that might seem very simple to other people often become a nightmare in the head of someone with AS. People with AS are often overly detail oriented and don't know how to arrange details. They often can't tell which details are important to pay attention to, and which they can ignore. Therefore, simple things can seem overwhelming. Sometimes, they just need someone to walk them through all the steps of something—how to cook, how to clean, or how to do other tasks. Because of these reasons, adults with AS can often benefit from support and guidance with everyday household tasks.

5. Reassurance and guidance

Adults with AS often have a high need for reassurance, and often just need someone they can ask questions of. If they do something enough times, they can often get the routine down enough to be able to do it independently, but it will take a few times, and new questions will sometimes pop up. Someone who can keep them on task and focused can really help. Also, sustaining attention on tasks is sometimes difficult. Distraction comes easily. Other things attract the person's attention, whether they be thoughts or objects or things they want to do.

Also, many adults with AS get sucked into obsessions; they might start playing video games, writing, doing crafts or working on something that maintains their focus for a long time, and they forget to eat or do other household chores. Reminders can be helpful at times like these.

6. Transportation

Many adults with AS do not drive. Driving involves a lot of multi-tasking abilities and ability to sustain attention on one thing, make decisions effectively under pressure, and be able to deal with a lot of sensory information at once. A lot of people with AS have difficulty in many of these areas. Some people with AS can take buses, but some areas do not have very good bus service. An individual's level of anxiety and functioning might prevent him from being able to effectively navigate a bus system. Transportation to doctors' appointments, shopping, and recreation, therefore, is a big need for many adults with AS.

7. Budgeting

Some adults with AS need help figuring out their budgeting; how to spend money appropriately; how to pay bills, when to pay bills and that sort of thing.

8. Errands

Many individuals with AS need help shopping and completing errands. Besides the transportation problem, some find stores too overwhelming to navigate on their own. Stores can be too loud, too much going on at once, lights too bright, or music too loud.

9. Nutrition

Some with AS need help to plan, develop and choose meals for themselves that will be nutritious, healthy, and somewhat balanced rather than eating chips and pizza for dinner—or whatever else they can find that is appealing and doesn't need much cooking.

10. Emotional Support

When you boil it all down, a lot of times adults with AS simply need some kind of emotional support. They live in a world that that does not seem secure or safe. All around them is chaos, people doing things in ways that they can't quite understand or that doesn't quite make sense to them. All around them people are expecting more of them then they often feel able to give or do. The rules seem foreign, and they always seem to be doing something wrong. It can make a person feel quite anxious or insecure to live in a world like this.

An adult with AS doesn't have the same ability to "take things for granted" that others do. They can't assume that "things are going to be all right," or that just because it worked one time or even five, that any given thing will work the next time. Therefore, it can be very helpful to an adult with AS to have emotional support—that is, to be able to talk out their worries with someone on a daily basis, and get reassurance for the things that they are worried about. This can help minimize other physical and mental issues that might develop as a result of the added stress of the worries. Also, this connection with others gives them a base of connection and support that makes them feel more secure and able to go into the world and do the things that they need to do.

One should remember that the needs of every adult with AS are very different, and the above described needs will not be true of every person with AS. Some adults will have some of them but not all of them; others will have very different needs. These are only the most common. Most needs can fit into these categories, but not all. It is important to assess the needs of the particular adult with AS before starting to make a services plan.

Executive Function and Mental Flexibility

One reason that those with Asperger's have challenges with many day-to-day activities is that many have deficits in two areas: executive function and mental flexibility.

Executive function—defined as "problems in areas such as planning, working memory, impulse control, inhibition and mental flexibility, and the initiation and monitoring of actions" (Trends in Cognitive Science, Jan 2004, "Executive Dysfunction in Autism)—is a major reason many adults with AS require a lot more help than you might think they would. The areas of the brain responsible for planning out activities, figuring out the steps, following the steps, following a sequence, are sometimes just not all there and individuals with AS can feel very lost.

Mental flexibility—the ability to figure out what to do if something goes wrong mid-activity, how to alter your plans to accommodate the problem, how to effectively problem solve, how to see alternate ways of getting something done—is often something people with AS have a huge problem with. It's not being stubborn or stupid; it's just the way their brain works.

What are some other needs that adults with AS have?

On an online message board, adults with Asperger's were talking about what they would ideally like to have help with if they had the chance.

One woman made a long list of things that she would like help with:

- Keeping on top of housework
- Getting out of the house on time
- Getting to places on time and without getting lost

- Getting dressed more quickly and easily

- Drinking enough—if I manage all the steps to get a drink without spilling it I forget to drink it

- Getting more work

- Get exercise regularly, I need it for physical and mental health

- Handling work—organizing all the stuff I need to do though I am posting letters

- Going to things that are distant or difficult in some way

- Keeping my car in working order

- Making phone calls to arrange things

- Coping if any important coping item (computer, phone, watch, etc.) does not work

- Explaining to people what my problems are and that they may seem nothing but are not

- Dealing with times when I have allowed myself to do nothing but sink into inertia then depression

Another middle aged woman made a similar list, which echoed some of the same themes:

- Cooking

- Cleaning

- Getting kids ready for school

- Maintaining routines

- Getting out of the house

- Organizing my possessions

- Monitoring my health and seeking medical attention when needed

- Talking to people
- Getting books out of the library and taking them back on time
- Doing university assignments
- Walking my dog
- Shopping
- Doing things with my kids
- Trying new things
- Getting off the computer
- Going to bed
- Hygiene
- Making meal plans
- Cleaning the cat litter and picking up dog poo
- Mowing the lawn
- Taking out the garbage
- Cleaning my car
- Applying for benefits
- Maintaining my car
- Maintaining my computers
- Buying, writing and sending cards
- Eating healthy food
- Laundry
- Leaving the house on time
- Making decisions
- Doing what I've planned
- Looking for employment or education opportunities

- Making phone calls

As you can see, adults with AS can need a LOT of support. This is not to say that every adult with AS has problems in all of these areas! Some have more difficulty with everyday issues than others. Most find ways to cope with their difficulties in these areas. They devise systems of doing the tasks that make them more feasible, they get a friend to help, or they might have a spouse or other family member to help. Most are able to do these tasks more or less, but not always consistently, and wish they had help to make the task not so onerous, or to help them do the tasks more consistently.

Personal care attendant (PCA)

So where does this leave us? We now know that adults with AS have a lot of needs for services, but where can you get them? A lot of these needs are the kind that can be fulfilled through a PCA, or personal care attendant. Sometimes insurance will pay for a PCA with certain disabilities or impairments, but they are most often physical and most do not cover autism as a qualifying condition. Some states are trying to pass laws mandating autism insurance, so that these services are more readily available.

State run Developmentally Disabled programs

The only real place to be able to obtain the services needed above is through Developmentally Disabled programs run by the state, but these often have stringent admission requirements and waiting lists that often run years. A lot of these programs only accept people who also have some level of mental retardation or otherwise low functioning. A lot of these programs also require you to have been shown to be disabled before the age of 18—or sometimes 21 or 22—which cuts out a large portion of adults with AS who were not diagnosed until adulthood. Sometimes one can get home health care services through Medicaid programs, but again, eligibility differs.

One young woman who called to inquire if she could get services through a local organization that provided services to people with developmental disabilities, such as Asperger's, was told, "If you're living on your own, you're already too high functioning to receive our services." To which she replied, "You think being able to use a computer all day and cook an occasional meal is high functioning?" The woman said, "Well, I certainly don't, but the state of New York does."

States do vary widely on the level of services they will provide, and to whom. The requirements you need to be eligible for services, the length of waiting lists, and other such things are different depending on the state.

Frustration with not being able to get services geared towards adults with Asperger's, who were high functioning but still in need of support, was a recent topic on the Asperger's Internet site Wrongplanet.net. User Belfast commented, "I live in the Northeast U.S. I know of no group (public or private) that deals (exclusively or primarily) with ASD dx'd (diagnosed) adults, esp. "high-functioning" people. All that exists seems to be for children or for those w/another co-occurring dx such as mental retardation. I'm cognitively quite "able", yet I'm not "NT" enough (or whatever one wishes to call it) to participate in everyday life.

It's so ridiculous that the powers that be seem to think we (individuals w/the dx) just "poof !" disappear at age 18 or 21…Not to mention, those of us who were never dx'd until already having reached adulthood—which is NOT proof that we don't need help, only that we made it this far without it & could really use some understanding & assistance, at long last."

User Fraya commented on the fact that most adults who are not diagnosed until after age 21 do not usually qualify for services, yet they are often the ones who need them the most: "If anything the ones who made it to adulthood before being diagnosed probably need help the most. I see a lot of disorders, self-image issues and post traumatic stress caused by growing up being a stranger in a strange and hostile land and not knowing why or being given any understanding or compassion."

Kids with AS grow into adults with AS

There seems to be a belief by many people that kids with AS will "outgrow" their problems if only given early intervention, and that is one reason a lot of programs and money is devoted to kids with AS. But kids with AS grow into adults with AS, and although it is important to help kids and teenagers develop as many coping skills and improve as much as they can while they are still young, few outgrow their symptoms enough to not need any help when they reach the age of 18 or 21.

There are still issues left over, and the lack of support for adults with AS is becoming a real problem as more and more kids with AS age out of the system and are left with no or little services to help them cope with life. User Krex speaks to this, "As to "out growing"...yeah, I have learned some coping skills but haven't heard from many adults with AS who don't still struggle with some AS traits and co-morbids as adults and I think that many of our strengths could benefit society if they would make a small investment in resources to help with some of the "problem areas". It seems, then, that the area of services for adults with AS is definitely something that needs improvement.

While it is true that it is hard to qualify for a lot of services offered, this is not to say that no one with AS will be able to get services. Again, it depends on your individual situation and case. You will need to apply with your state to see if you can qualify or not. A good caseworker, often supplied by mental health agencies, can help you navigate the system. If you do qualify for services, there is a lot you can get that can increase your quality of life quite a bit. Let's look at some of the services available.

State Organizations

All states have offices that deal with people who have developmental disabilities. These offices are often joint with offices for the mentally retarded or the elderly. You need to go through an application process in order to get these services. You will need extensive documentation from all the doctors, psychiatrists and psychologists you have seen attesting to your disability. A social history, psychosocial report, and other tests such as measures of your intellectual and adaptive behavior will be required. Such tests include things like the Leiter International Performance Scale, Adaptive Behavior Assessment System, Scales of Independent Behavior and so on are often used. You usually need proof you were disabled before a certain age, which is different for every state. Intelligence tests are also needed and often your IQ determines whether or not you are eligible for services; many states do not have the resources to provide services for people with higher than a certain IQ (intelligence quotient).

If you do get accepted, you will be eligible for a variety of services, depending on your needs. These will be determined by the office, you, and your caseworker. Such services usually include:

1. **Employment Services**: Vocational training, counseling, job placement help, job coaches, and technological aids that help with a person being able to perform a job. Transportation to a job is often given as well.

136

2. **In home health care**: aides to come to your house and help you with activities of daily living, such as cooking, cleaning, recreation, shopping, and whatever else you might need.

3. **Supported living services**: extra help to help you live independently in your house; varies according to your needs

4. **Other housing support**: could be group homes, supported living placements, etc.

5. **Crisis intervention**: helps with short term emergencies

6. **Counseling**: free of charge to you

7. **Some states offer adaptive equipment or environmental modifications**; if you need your living space sound-proofed due to sensory issues, for example, or needed other accommodations due to your disability, the agency would help provide it if it deemed the need medically necessary.

8. **Help with budgeting and finances**: this could include training on how to manage daily household finances or how to ensure bills are paid on time.

9. **Transportation**: such as to medical appointments, shopping and recreational activities

10. **Respite care**: if your normal caretaker is not available, another one will often be supplied

11. **Service coordination**: help you gain access to the services you need to help you achieve your goals

It seems, then, that if you can access services through the department of developmental disabilities in your state, they can be quite helpful.

Example of what one state does to serve adults with disabilities

The state of Oregon seems to have one of the more comprehensive programs in the country for adults with disabilities, including adults with Asperger's. They utilize something called a brokerage program. The adult gets to choose what services they want to receive and who they want to hire to receive these services. They get allotted a certain budget to do this. The goal of these services is to give the adult as much independence and self determination as possible.

The State of Oregon website, says that, "Brokerage Support Services are in-home or other personal supports that assist an individual to live in their own home or with family or friends and to fully participate in community life, including work. Support services are based upon people having choice and control over life goals and services. Each individual will receive an individual plan and will be able to select and monitor the providers of desired services." (http://www.oregon.gov/DHS/dd/adults/supports.shtml)

The website further describes what is needed to be eligible for services:

- Must have its origin in the brain

- Must be established prior to the age of 22, or in the case of mental retardation the condition must be determined before 18 years of age

- Must be expected to last indefinitely

- Must result in significant impairments in at least two areas of daily functioning: self care, communication, cognitive, mobility, self direction, capacity for independent living and economic self sufficiency

- The impairments must not be primarily related to: mental illness, substance abuse, an emotional disorder, Attention Deficit/Hyperactivity Disorder (ADHD), a learning disability or sensory impairment.

Services available in Oregon: Example

As we discussed, services vary by state but examining the policies of one state can give us an idea of what is available nationally. Oregon has quite a long list of services available to those who qualify. Among those are:

- Chore services—help with household cleaning tasks that no one in the household is able to do

- Community inclusion supports—help the person maintain ties to and participate in the community; help maintain physical and mental skills; provide instruction in skills the person wants to learn

- Community living skills:

- Personal skills—such as eating, personal hygiene, bathing, dressing, and mobility

- Socialization—development of interpersonal interaction skills

- Communication—helping the person to use or improve expressive and receptive communication skills

- Personal environment skills—cooking, laundry, planning and preparing meals, budgeting

- Family training skills—provides training to family on how to better care or support the person with a disability

- Homemaker skills—general household activities

- Occupational therapy

- Physical therapy

- Special diet—will pay for special food deemed medically necessary to sustain the person; for example, gluten free foods, or supplements that the person needs to take for their health.

Oregon gets creative in what they will offer and gives the individual a lot of choice in what kind of services they feel they will most benefit from. One adult with Asperger's in Bend, Oregon said that her personal care aide cooked with her, shopped with her, helped her with budgeting and took her on walks. She found it very helpful to have this person help her to get these tasks done. Another woman with AS, also in Bend, said that she wasn't accepted into the brokerage program with people for developmental disabilities, but was able to find someone to help her access services and get an aide through the mental health department. A good caseworker will be aware of all the programs you can apply for and try to get you services through any avenue available.

Private organizations

There are also many private organizations available that cater to people with disabilities. A lot of these services are paid for by Medicaid or certain state agencies. If you have Medicaid, you will have a much better chance of having services like these paid for. A caseworker will know agencies in your individual state that can help fund these programs, or the people running the program will.

Programs like this often have the following components:

- They often run sheltered workshops or have other employment opportunities for the people they serve

- They help with housing

- They help transportation

- Provide social activities and recreation

For example, the organization *Opportunity Resources* in Missoula, Montana offers the following employment opportunities to people with disabilities, including Asperger's, that need a little more support:

- Packaging and Assembly

- Document destruction

- Wood Products (building wood products)

- Farming jobs on a ranch

- Various supported work crews

Opportunity Resources (www.opportunityresources.com) also offers day programs to fill its clients' time with enriching activities: "We have a day program for persons with Developmental Disabilities that enhances their quality of life. By choosing recreational and social activities, our consumers learn to make better use of their downtime when they are not in production jobs at ORI. We offer art classes, enrichment activities in the community, exercise programs, and the opportunity for individuals served to have social interaction with their peers. Our consumers take part in outings like trips to the library, the humane society, music classes, the Rocky Mountain Elk Foundation, museums, as well as other outdoor activities that address their need for physical health. We offer board games, movies, current event groups, men's group, dart team, spiritual enrichment class and computer access to provide opportunities for social interaction."

This organization also offers group homes and supported living for people in apartments, where people live alone but have access to a support staff person with any questions or problems that might arise 24 hours a day.

Case management to help coordinate services, as well as counseling services, is also available.

If you look at the programs offered by other private organizations, you will usually see a similar array of services offered. Supported employment, residential support, recreation, transportation and case management are usually standard. However, these organizations have their own entrance requirements as well, and you usually have to be pretty low functioning to gain services; plus, there are long wait lists.

Other Ideas: Paying Privately, or Bartering

So, when it comes down to it, these things are good if you can get them, but not everyone can. You can always hire someone privately to get the help you need, but most people with AS do not have the money for this. Sometimes family helps out with this, and sometimes they are not able to.

One idea that might work in some towns who have this program is to utilize a local time dollar program. A time dollar program is a rather creative new form of currency that is popping up in many cities across the country. People donate their skills to other people—whatever it might be, if you're good at the guitar and want to give guitar lessons, and someone else is good at cooking, you would trade an hour of guitar lessons for an hour of cooking. If you were good at babysitting and someone else was good at massage, you could baby-sit for an hour in order to get a massage. It doesn't have to be from the same person, either; people sign up, and their interests and abilities are put into a database of people. When you spend an hour doing something for one person, you can then take your credit from that and ask another person in the system to do something for you. This would work well for people with Asperger's because they often have specialized interests and skills that they might not be able to translate into a full or even part time job, but could definitely do on an occasional or even regular basis for someone else. In turn, they could get help cooking, cleaning, with transportation, or with any of the other things that they needed help with.

Not all cities have this, but many do; one example is Portland, Maine. The *Hour Exchange* in Portland is a great example of a time dollar program that has been going on a long time. Located at www.hourexchangeportland.org, their website gives many tips for how such a program works and ideas for how a person could set such a program up in their own community. The *Hour Exchange* believes that all people have something to give; everyone can do something. This theory is especially helpful for adults with Asperger's whose strengths and weaknesses might be especially uneven. The speaker Wolf Dunaway, an adult with autism who often speaks at various events around the country, once told the following story at a speech: "Everyone can do something. Can't do anything but tear pieces of paper into little pieces? You can get a job as a document shredder for a few hours a week." This anecdote reminds us that no matter how much trouble someone might seem to have in functioning in the world, with the right supports, and matching a job to their interests and abilities, everyone truly can do something.

The philosophy of the *Hour Exchange* aligns with this as well:

"Our Mission: Hour Exchange Portland is a service exchange based on Time, the currency of equality that empowers individuals to utilize their assets and enhance their lives, neighborhood and community.

Assets: We are all assets. Every human being has something of value to contribute.

Equality: At the heart of every time exchange is equality. One hour of service equals one Time Dollar, regardless of the service. All people are valued equally.

Reciprocity: Helping works better as a two way street. The question, "How can I help you?" needs to be changed to, "How can we help each other build the world we both want to live in?"

Redefining Work: Work is beyond price. Work must be redefined to include all of the activities it takes to sustain families, neighborhoods and communities, to help democracy work and to advance social justice. This kind of work needs to be honored.

Social Networks: We need each other. Networks are stronger than individuals. People can help each other build communities of support, strength and trusting relationships.

Respect: Everyone matters. We must respect where people are in the moment, not where we hope they will be at some future point." (www.hourexchangeportland.org)

Everyone is an asset in some way to someone else. We just need to figure out what someone is good at. Everyone can do something. And if you can help another person out, then first, you feel good about yourself—which is a powerful antidepressant; and second, at least in this program, helping someone else means you can start to get some of the help and support you need for yourself. When it all comes down to it, this is the very meaning of being part of a community; people helping other people with what they have and what they can do.

It would be great if there were more programs like this. Perhaps in time, when word gets around, people will hear about them and start their own time dollar program in their own community.

Of course, one does not need a formal program to arrange a bartering arrangement per se; but it is a lot harder to find people to barter with otherwise. If you know someone who might be in need of a skill that you possess, though, and you think they can help you out as well, it might be something worth trying.

Independent Living Centers

Independent living centers (ILCs) are community based organizations that try to help people with disabilities meet their daily needs in the most respectful way possible. They provide services and advocacy for people in need of it, and try to maximize the potential of people with disabilities to do whatever they want or need to do. The services provided by ILCs vary widely by city. Usually, they offer some kind of advocacy, independent living skills training, information and referral services, and peer counseling. Independent living centers can help you get connected with the services you need. They can help you figure out what you are eligible for, and how to get it.

The official definition of an independent living center is as follows from Section 702 of the Rehabilitation Act of 1973, "The term 'center for independent living' means a consumer-controlled, community-based, cross-disability, non-residential private nonprofit agency that is designed and operated within a local community by individuals with disabilities and provides an array of independent living services."

(http://www.bcm.edu/ilru/html/publications/directory/index .html)

Independent living centers are based on the following three theories, according to "A Center for Independent Living History," (http://www.ilusa.com/articles/021300CILHistoryZukas.html):

1. Those who know best the needs of disabled people and how to meet those needs are the disabled people themselves.

2. The needs of the disabled can be met most effectively by comprehensive programs which provide a variety of services.

3. Disabled people should be integrated fully into their community.

ILCs can be a very useful resource to people with disabilities. You can do an Internet search for your local center or call local government offices for more information about your local ILC.

Other Services fitting More Basic Needs of Adults with AS

Besides all the organizations working to fit the needs of people with AS and other disabilities, there are organizations that also exist to fill other, more basic needs you might have.

Food stamps

If you make below a certain income level, then you are eligible for food stamps. Food stamps can help you purchase food for the month. Instead of actual stamps, like they used to do, you will get an electronic debit card that you can use at most major food retailers to buy food. Some farmers' markets even accept them. A certain amount is put on your card once a month. The amount differs quite a bit from state to state, and it also depends on how much income you have, and how many people are in your household. If you have kids or more people, you will get more money. Amounts generally range between $1-200 a month for a single person, but again, it varies.

To apply for food stamps, you need to figure out what the appropriate government office is to call (sometimes if you do a Google search for the words "food stamps" and your county and state, this information can be obtained pretty easily; or sometimes the phone number can be found in the front of the local phone book, or by calling Department of Human Services in your city, who can then refer you to the right place). You then have to fill out an application and go in for an interview. A decision will usually be made within 30 days about whether you are eligible to get food stamps or not. If your situation is really dire and you have no food or money, you can apply to get emergency food stamps within five days.

Section 8 Housing

If you need assistance with paying for rental housing, you can apply for a Section 8 Housing voucher. The waiting lists for these vouchers are usually quite long, unfortunately, so you should apply as soon as you know you might need help, and be prepared to wait. If approved, though, these vouchers can help a lot in your housing search. Another thing to look for to help pay for housing costs are apartment buildings that have their own subsidies attached. These are apartments where if you qualify, you will only have to pay a certain percentage of your income to live there.

Medicare and Medicaid

Both of these programs are national health insurance programs that can help you pay for health insurance if you are either very low income, disabled, or both. Most people who receive disability payments usually get health insurance as well through one of these programs. This can help you pay for your doctors' visits, prescription medications, and any hospital stays that you have.

Social security benefits

Many people with autism spectrum disorders are eligible for disability benefits; a certain amount of money that is paid to them every month. This usually differs per person and situation. Some people get SSI, Supplemental Security Income, which is a smaller amount of money used to offset living expenses. Others can get SSDI, Social Security Disability Income, which is usually a larger amount. Generally, the more you have worked, the more you are eligible to get. This can be a good supplement for a person with Asperger's who has difficulty securing and maintaining employment to have. It can provide at least some form of an independent life.

When You Have Other Medical Needs Besides Asperger's

We all know that when you have a disability, it doesn't automatically preclude you from having other medical issues too. In other words, you may have Asperger's, yes, but you may also have bipolar disorder, severe anxiety, and Crohn's disease, high blood pressure, whatever. You need to find a way to treat all of your medical problems. Sometimes it can be hard to figure out where to go for help, or even what kind of help you need. Sometimes it can be hard to tell what problems are part of Asperger's and what are part of other illnesses that might require different treatment. People with AS, for example, can often have ADD and depression as well; these have different treatments than AS. You might say, "Oh, I get angry so easily because of my Asperger's, so I can't do much about it," but you should stop and think if there are any other causes that can be addressed, most likely through therapy.

If you need help with other mental health issues, contact your local mental health department and ask for an evaluation through them. Most cities have low cost community mental health counseling centers that can help if you don't have much money. Most cities also have low cost medical clinics you can go to if you don't have health insurance or a way to pay for medical care. Some cities have a hotline for local social services called 211, where you can dial and tell the person who answers what kind of help you need—and they will tell you what social agency to go to for it. Not all cities have this, but many do. To see if your city has 211 services, simply dial the number in any phone and see if it works.

The point is, if you have other medical needs, either psychological or physical, there are community services designed to help you access care for these issues if you cannot do it on your own. It is important to care of yourself and all of your needs.

Final Thoughts

Adults with Asperger's have a very complex set of needs. They need support and direction in many areas. They often need instruction on how to do tasks the rest of the world might take for granted. They may need assistance with housing and other basic needs. There are many local and state programs in existence to help with these needs, but they are hard for many with AS to access due to eligibility requirements and limited funding. With any hope, these services will be expanded in the future to fill the very real need that adults with Asperger's have for support. Still, a dedicated and creative person can find the help they need in the community; from all of the ideas presented here, it is possible to pick and choose different things to find the help you need.

6. How and when do I tell people I have Asperger's?

The issue of when and how to tell someone you have Asperger's—if at all—is not simple. Disclosing this to a close loved one, a friend, a family member, your boss, or simply the mail man is called self-disclosure. Simply put, the term self-disclosure refers to when you tell someone that you have Asperger's, and when you don't. There are certain times when it is not necessary, sometimes when it should probably be avoided, and other times when it is imperative. There are times when you need to stick up for yourself and your rights as a person with Asperger's, or any other autistic spectrum disorder. There are certain rights you have that need to be respected. You have the right to have your needs, thoughts and feelings respected, whether you have Asperger's or not. In this chapter, we will talk about when to bring Asperger's into the picture, and how to stand up for what you need. When you talk about self-advocacy, you also need to talk about the neurodiversity movement, which will be explored later on.

Should You Tell People You Have Asperger's?

As we just mentioned, one important part of knowing about Asperger's is knowing when this information needs to be shared and when it would be better not to. Questions will come up, such as... Who do I tell? How many people? Do I tell just my close friends, or everyone? Do I tell my boss at work, or just a few select co-workers that I trust? Do I need to tell my professors? How much about Asperger's do I need to share? Or should I just keep it to myself and not tell anyone?

Why is this decision important?

Telling someone you have Asperger's syndrome is a lot more significant than, say, telling them what you had for lunch that day, or that your kid won the state spelling bee. It can be a very stigmatizing thing. People have a lot of strange perceptions about autism, and about illness or "syndromes" of any kind.

They can be very judgmental about anyone who is different. The average member of the public knows very little to nothing about autism and even less about Asperger's. If you mention autism, the only image they might have in their head is the guy in *Rain Man* rocking back and forth in the corner. If you mention Asperger's, you'll probably get a blank stare. If you then go on to mention that it's either a kind of autism or a high functioning form of autism, again, you will be back to the *Rain Man* thing.

Some people may be scared by this information. They may feel they do not know how to interact with you, or do not want to put the energy and effort into figuring out how to interact with you.

Not knowing much about autism or Asperger's, they may even be scared that you will be dangerous or violent. Some people lump all mental illnesses together—not that Asperger's is a mental illness but sometimes people who do not know better will see it as that—and think of everyone who is different as someone to treat with kid gloves or else run the opposite way from.

It is hard to tell in advance how someone will react

Not everyone will react this way. Some will be genuinely glad and pleased you felt comfortable enough to share this information with them. They will be glad to finally have a better understanding of you, and how to help you. They may have noticed a few things were "off" about the way you interacted with them, but didn't want to bring it up without seeming rude. This gives them the opportunity to ask questions and learn about how to better interact with you. This may bring you closer, sharing this knowledge with them. This is a good scenario, because you will have improved your relations with people who react in this way. They will know now, for example, if you say something that comes off as a little rude, that you didn't mean to be rude but simply didn't know how else to say it. If you leave the room abruptly because you need a sensory break, they will understand. If you lose the words and can't think of how to tell a co-worker something, they can act as an ally and interpret for you. If you need help understanding a social situation, a good ally in the workplace or anywhere else can be invaluable. There are many reasons that self-disclosure of Asperger's can have a positive effect. It is hard to tell ahead of time what the result will be, so that is one reason it is good to start small.

Four Reasons to Disclose Asperger's Syndrome

1. To Improve Your Relationships

You should disclose Asperger's syndrome if you feel it will help a relationship—either with a friend, loved one or co-worker. If you feel this will help these people to understand you on a deeper level and see your quirks as a symptom of your neurology instead of willfulness or deliberately trying to be stubborn, then it might be a good idea to let them know.

2. To Gain Accommodations

If there are things you need accommodations for, such as a quieter workspace, written instructions, a more explicit communication style, etc, in the workplace, then you should disclose this need and the diagnosis that caused it.

3. To Make You Feel More Whole

If disclosing Asperger's makes you feel more whole as a person—in other words, if you want people to see ALL of you, and you feel this is an important part of you that you want respected and acknowledged by others, you might choose to disclose.

4. Societal Reasons

Each person you tell about Asperger's is one more person who learns what it really is, and brings this knowledge to share with the rest of the world. They gain a more accurate idea of what Asperger's looks like, rather than what is presented in the media.

Stephen Shore talks about this in his December 2002 *Autism Asperger's Digest* magazine article, "Disclosure for People on the Autism Spectrum: Working Towards a Better Mutual Understanding." Stephen says, "Each individual disclosure works, one person at a time, towards changing the still-common societal description of a person on the autism spectrum being only the nonverbal, antisocial, self-abusive child flapping his hands in the corner. Effective disclosure helps a partner, a job supervisor, or a family member better understand all that makes up autism. With this understanding, they come to see us as people capable of contributing to society, sometimes in significant ways. The second effect of disclosure relates to society has a whole. Each disclosure about autism that results in this deeper mutual understanding changes not only the disclosee's construct of the disorder but potentially everyone else with whom the disclosee comes in contact. In some situations, these people can become ambassadors, passing along their new understanding to others."

Four Reasons Not To Disclose Asperger's Syndrome

1. Possible Negative Repercussions on Relationships

If this information will have a negative effect on your relationship, then you should not disclose it. If it will cause someone to doubt your abilities or think of you as less of a person, then it is not a good idea. Especially if you know the person does not have much understanding of disability issues or is prejudiced against people with disabilities, you should not disclose.

2. Casual Relationships

If the person is not someone you have regular contact with, or someone who is not very important in your life, then it is not important to disclose. For example, the mailman or someone who works in a shop does not need to know.

3. If It's Not Broke, Don't Fix It

If things seem to be going well in the workplace, and you have no need for any accommodations, then there is probably no reason to disclose.

4. You're Not Comfortable Disclosing

If you simply do not feel comfortable telling a certain person or group of people, then don't. Not everyone needs to know. A general rule of thumb is to only tell people you feel comfortable with and trust to some degree.

Stephen Shore continues to discuss the issue of disclosure by mentioning work by Liane Holiday Willey: "*In Pretending to Be Normal: Living with Asperger's Syndrome* (Willey, 1999), author Liane Holiday Willey describes three groups of people to whom disclosure can be made. The first group consists of people who need to know. These are people with whom the person has regular direct contact in such a way that interactions with them are affected by autism. … However, disclosure may be inappropriate if the information is irrelevant or will have a negative impact on the relationship. … The second group consists of people with whom there is frequent contact, including family members, friends, classmates, or teachers, but not enough regularity that the autism might create a problem between them. The third group consists of people who do not need to know about the disorder. This might include the postman, neighbors, the cashier at the corner store, and acquaintances."

In the end, then, the decision whether to disclose or not should be made on a potential calculation on what the impact will be on the relationship. Is this person likely to see this positively or negatively? How relevant is it to the situation?

When to disclose?

Generally, you should disclose if you are in a situation where something is not going well, and this information about your diagnosis would hopefully smooth things over and improve the situation. You should ask for a meeting, with co-workers, your boss, or so on rather than just blurt it out.

What information should be disclosed?

If you are in a workplace, try to keep the information relevant to the difficulties that Asperger's causes you in that environment. For example, if you needed to be moved to a quieter area, you would mention that Asperger's causes some sensory issues like sensitivity to sound, and that moving to a quieter area would help. You wouldn't discuss, for example, how you just can't stand the feeling of seams in socks, because it wouldn't be relevant to the discussion or your duties at your job. You also don't need to go into the history of Asperger's or give anything that does not relate to how you perform your job.

For family or friends, disclose as much or as little as you feel comfortable with. Tell them how Asperger's affects you, how it makes you feel, how it alters your experience of life. Ask for help in areas that you have problems with if you feel comfortable doing so. There is nothing you have to tell them, but on the other hand, hopefully they will want to hear a lot about it and learn how it affects your life. Only you can gauge how much you feel is okay to share; you can start with a little information and give more as time goes on if this makes you feel better about it.

A Note About Shame

Different people have different ideas and feelings about an Asperger's diagnosis. Some people feel very ashamed and don't want anyone to know. They can't imagine why you would ever want to tell anyone. As far as they're concerned, it's their problem, and they're going to keep it to themselves. No one else needs to know. Others are relieved and set free by the diagnosis. They gain a sense of pride in themselves after learning about the reasons why they struggle with certain areas. They gain a sense of self-acceptance. They realize that along with certain challenges, Asperger's also brings many strengths, such as the ability to focus on things for long periods of time, out of the box thinking, different ways and approaches of doing things that often get the job done better than their typical peers.

They realize that the world is made up of many, many different types of people, and if it weren't, half the things we rely on an everyday basis would not have been invented. The world, in a sense, needs people with different abilities and difficulties to be well balanced; the world needs the strengths of everyone, not just a select few. They choose to have a sense of pride about their difference.

The Neurodiversity Movement

The neurodiversity movement was born out of these realizations. In its most simple definition, the neurodiversity movement is about recognizing that it's okay to be different. On his blog "Spectrum Siblings," at http://frogger11758.wordpress.com, a young man by the name of Cale defines it this way: "Neurodiversity is the belief that there is a wide range of ways that the brain can be organized. None of these particular ways are any better or any worse than the other varieties, merely different." The website Neurodiversity.com has the slogan, "Honoring the Diversity of Human Wiring." It lists hundreds and hundreds of links related to all things autism and Asperger's. There are many, many different definitions of neurodiversity. People will use it to mean many different things. Basically, though, what follows is the most commonly accepted meaning of the term.

One by one, a whole community of autistic and Asperger's people came together, bonded by the following realizations.

1. We are not broken. There is no reason to fix us. Yes, we think differently than others, but that is not an

2. We deserve respect. Just because we think differently and act differently than others does not mean that we should be treated as less then. Our nervous systems might get overwhelmed more easily than others; we may need to pace, flap, or fidget to calm ourselves; we may have trouble speaking at times or not speak at all; or we may go on for way too long about an interest that we have. So what? Some people have blue eyes, some have brown eyes; the way people's brains work should be accorded the same respect.

3. We do not need to be cured. Autism and Asperger's are not diseases. They are different ways of thinking. If you develop a way to screen us out at birth (as some scientists and major autism organizations are attempting to do), you will eradicate a whole population with skills and abilities essential to our culture that cannot be replaced. If you erase autism, you eradicate a whole way of being.

It probably does not need to be said that the last principle has been met with quite a bit of resistance from many in the autism community. The autism community is largely divided by parents with autistic kids or adults (including those with Asperger's) who think that autism is a horrible thing and has robbed their child of a meaningful, functional life; and those adults with Asperger's or high functioning autism who resent being portrayed in such a negative way and are starting to try to get the message out that autism is not a bad thing. One can see both sides of this battle; the severity of autism spectrum disorders vary widely, and one might say it is not exactly fair to compare those with what we would call lower functioning autism and very few traditional prospects in life with those with Asperger's who can hold down a job but have difficulty with social appropriateness or sensory overload at times.

Along this debate, there are people who feel these tenets are important to very different degrees, of course. Some adults feel, yes, it is important to respect our positive traits, but they don't get angry over the idea of a cure; some feel that yes, they have so many difficulties and problems with many areas of life that they would like to be cured if there was such a thing available. Others are appalled at the idea. Parents fall along the same lines: some think their kids are fine the way they are, others wish for more. Some see it as a disease, and some see it as a difference; and most fall somewhere in between the two.

The most important thing the neurodiversity community has in common, though, is the sense of autism as something to be celebrated and something to be proud of. The autism community of adults with Asperger's and autism is a very strong one. It flourishes online in email groups and message boards devoted to discussing Asperger's issues.

Some are groups devoted to daily living issues, and some are more political, discussing ways to make the general public more aware of what they feel are more accurate, positive images of people with autism and Asperger's. They write letters, speak at conferences and at committees, educate their school boards, teachers, and local schools. They come out as autistic to their jobs and communities in an attempt to spread the word that the face of autism and Asperger's can be a lot more positive than you think. That people with Asperger's are an important part of their communities. That they can be loyal, helpful, dedicated, creative problem solvers. That they matter. They advocate for accommodations where needed and more understanding of the difficulties in Asperger's. In short, they work for something known as self-advocacy—the ability to advocate on your own behalf.

7. Self Advocacy

Self advocacy is the ability to effectively communicate, negotiate and assert your own needs, and take steps to get them met. People with Asperger's need to learn how to advocate for themselves in order to be able to better function in the world around them.

A young woman with Asperger's by the name of Katie Miller has taken the lead in advocating for herself and the community of those with autism and Asperger's. When the organization Autism Speaks posted a video with a very negative message about autism called "I Am Autism"— talking in a gloomy, dismal voice about destroying lives, preventing people from ever being happy, destroying marriage, bankrupting families, and so on—she wrote her own video with a script based largely on the script of the Autism Speaks video. In part, the transcript reads like this:

"We are the Autistic Community. We are from all nations, all faiths, all languages. We search for acceptance, dignity, respect, compassion, and tolerance. We want a place in the community, an education, a high quality of life, and to make choices about our own lives. We want our voices to be heard and to contribute to a growing awareness you never anticipated. We have challenges, but we are equal in our humanity. We speak the only language that matters: support for one another. Our capacity to love is greater than your capacity to overwhelm. Hatred is naïve. You are alone. We are a community of Autistic People. We have a voice. We speak, type, point, sing, flap, and squeal. You think that because some of us cannot speak, that we have nothing to say."

In effect, it is an anthem for a community, calling on all its members and the general public to realize and respect the voices of those with autism, rather than to marginalize and ignore them.

Organizations Dedicated to Self Advocacy

One of the largest, if not the largest, organizations devoted to self advocacy is called the Autistic Self Advocacy Network, or ASAN. It was started only a few years ago by a college student and a graduate student both on the autism spectrum, both with Asperger's. Ari Ne'eam and Scott Robertson did not like the negative messages about autism they were hearing in the media. They didn't like the negative assumptions people had when they heard about autism or Asperger's, or the lack of general awareness. They thought that people with Asperger's and autism should be able to speak up for themselves and their needs. Horrified by stories of teachers throwing autistic students in closets for punishment for acting out, of negative media attention and very little understanding of how to meet the needs of adults with Asperger's in the general public, the two started ASAN.

ASAN's slogan is "Nothing About Us, Without Us." They seek to get autistic adults engaged in the discussion of autism policy and services. They seek to organize community. Adults with Asperger's have many needs that are not being well served by present community services. Most organizations assume if you're not severely autistic and nonverbal, you don't need any help at all—this is not true. Adults with Asperger's can be valuable parts of the community, but need to be able to advocate for their needs to be able to do so. They need to be able to state their needs and work towards changing public and local policy to achieve this goal.

ASAN, according to its website at: www.autisticadvocacy.org, is…

"A non-profit organization run by and for autistic people. Our activities include public policy advocacy, community engagement to encourage inclusion and respect for neurodiversity, quality of life oriented research and the development of autistic cultural activities and other opportunities for autistic people to engage with others on the spectrum."

Its mission statement says that, "The Autistic Self Advocacy Network seeks to advance the principles of the disability rights movement in the world of autism. Drawing on the principles of the cross-disability community on issues such as inclusive education, community living supports and others, ASAN seeks to organize the community of Autistic adults and youth to have our voices heard in the national conversation about us. In addition, ASAN seeks to advance the idea of neurological diversity, putting forward the concept that the goal of autism advocacy should not be a world without Autistic people. Instead, it should be a world in which Autistic people enjoy the same access, rights and opportunities as all other citizens. Working in fields such as public policy, media representation, research and systems change, ASAN hopes to empower Autistic people across the world to take control of their own lives and the future of our common community. Nothing About Us, Without Us!"

ASAN has chapters in about a dozen different states and areas, and is based out of Washington, DC. Founder Ari Ne'eam, who was only a freshman in college when he started ASAN, has received national media attention for his efforts.

Newsweek explained Ari's goal well in a May 2009 article on him, called "Could A Gene Test Change Autism?" "The task he has taken on is daunting and controversial: he wants to change the way the world views autism. Autism is not a medical mystery that needs solving, he argues. It's a disability, yes, but it's also a different way of being, and "neurodiversity" should be accepted by society. Autistic people (he prefers this wording to "people with autism," a term many parents use, because he considers the condition intrinsic to a person's makeup) must be accommodated in the classroom and workplace and helped to live independently as adults—and he is pushing to make this happen for everyone on the spectrum. They should also be listened to. "We're having a national conversation about autism without the voices of people who should be at the center of that conversation," he says."

To this end, Ari and his organization have taken on some rather large organizations in their efforts to improve the public image of autism. When New York University's Child Development Center ran a campaign called "Ransom Notes" that featured messages like: "We have your child. We will make sure he lives a life full of isolation and is unable to ever take care of himself," ASAN took a major stand against the campaign and the scare tactics used. ASAN started a letter writing campaign and was able to successfully apply enough pressure on NYU to get them to pull the ad campaign. Ne'eam says, "There's a misperception that autism is some thief in the night that takes a normal child and places an autistic child in its place," he says. "That's not true." When another organization ran similar ads in Pennsylvania, ASAN once again came to the forefront to raise awareness of the ads and their inaccurate messages and the campaign was pulled.

Other Organizations

Some organizations such as Autism Speaks are trying to find a cure for autism and develop prenatal screening tests for autism. Some autistic and Asperger's adults are worried that this will take away a whole segment of a population that has skills and talents needed in the world. They feel devalued. And they are letting the world know. "But autism isn't a fatal condition. Should people without the disorder be allowed to judge the quality of life of someone who has it? "That is a message that the world doesn't want us here," says Ne'eam, "and it devalues our lives." (Newsweek May 2009).

The autism cure issue is not the only issue ASAN has with Autism Speaks. Autism Speaks, they maintain, has a history of putting out fear-mongering videos that prey on parents' anxieties and fears in hopes of getting donations. They take issue with a video Autism Speaks produced featuring a woman who stated that she had thought about driving off a bridge with her autistic daughter, and that the only reason she didn't is because her typical child needed her. They take issue with a more recent video called "I am Autism," which talks about destroying the lives of those touched with autism. The video proclaims, "I am autism. I have no interest in right or wrong. I will plot to rob you of your children and your dreams... And if you're happily married, I will make sure that your marriage fails. Your money will fall into my hands, and I will bankrupt you for my own self-gain." Sixty autism advocacy organizations, from the Arc of the United States, to the Bazelon Mental Health Law Center, the National Council on Independent Living, to many state and local self-advocacy groups such as the Michigan Disability Rights Coalition and the Green Mountain Self-Advocates in Vermont, came together to condemn Autism Speaks for their message of gloom and doom and dismal portrayal of autism.

Ne'eam states, "Contrary to the "I am Autism" video, which equates autism with AIDS and Cancer, autism is not a terminal disease. It is a disability, one that comes with significant challenges in a wide variety of realms. Yet the answer to those challenges is not to create a world in which people are afraid of people on the autism spectrum. The answer is not to create a world in which the word autism is met with terror, hatred and prejudice. It is to work to create a society that recognizes the civil rights of Autistic people and others with disabilities. It is to work to create a world in which people with disabilities can benefit from the supports, the services and the educational tools necessary to empower them to be full citizens in society."

These are the principles the self-advocacy movement was founded on. ASAN may be the biggest organization representing these principles for adults with Asperger's, but there are many smaller organizations local to different states and cities that you can find with a Google search. For information on finding a local ASAN chapter, see their website at www.autisticadvocacy.com. ASAN also maintains an active online presence, and a busy email list-serv where people come from all over to talk about Asperger's representation and advocacy.

There are other definitions of self-advocacy that don't involve so many political actions. Self Advocates As Leaders, a group based in Portland, Oregon, states on their website (http://www.asksaal.org) that:

All people should be able to speak up for themselves and make their own decisions and mistakes.

All people should be able to choose their own lifestyle and have control over their own things.

All people should work together as a team.

All people should have the right to choose an action and accept the consequences.

People First, another Oregon based disability organization at http://www.people1.org, states it even more simply by saying, "We want others to know that we are people first, and our disabilities come second."

Being your own self-advocate

But again, self-advocacy and appreciating neurodiversity does not always mean being political and taking stances against major organizations. There are many actions you can do in your everyday life to self-advocate for yourself.

If you are in a situation and you are getting overwhelmed, realizing this and asking for a break or to leave for a few minutes—it might seem simple but it is a vital skill to have, and a form of self-advocacy.

If you receive social services such as case management, and have someone come in to your house to help you with cleaning, cooking or other tasks; and you are not happy with the quality of services you are getting, or are being neglected in some way, speaking out is a form of self-advocacy. If your caseworker criticizes you or refuses to assist you in ways that have already been agreed on, and your report her to the agency you work with, that is self-advocacy; taking control of your life and what you need.

If someone sees you flapping your arms in a store and curses at you or shuns you, and you calmly and politely but firmly tell them, "I have Asperger's and I do this to relieve stress," you are standing up for yourself and helping to raise awareness of Asperger's and autism.

If you ask for extra time on tests in college, a less noisy atmosphere at work, or so on, you are advocating for yourself. It is not about trying to get the world changed to fit your every need, as some may accuse; it is not about being selfish; it is about having an even playing field, and having the world be accessible enough for you to function in it. You deserve at least that.

Part Two: Learning to Advocate for Yourself: A First Person Account

Sometimes, in everyday life, you go about your day not paying that much attention to your differences, and not wanting to share them with others. This is good, because the goal of an independent life is to, well, work around your differences to a point where they are not the focus of every day. You often make little accommodations for ourselves to get through the day—people with and without autism do this. You might take sensory breaks when you need them, make excuses to leave early if overwhelmed, bring headphones to a noisy environment, and so on. All perfectly good things.

But the problem comes when someone takes issue with your right to make minor accommodations to your environment in order to cope. Asperger's presents many sensory challenges and often you need to take a time out from what you are doing.

Sometimes, people will not understand this and can make your life quite difficult because of it. They will challenge your right to be able to make these accommodations for yourself. When this happens, it is time to step up and stick up for yourself. It is time to educate people, it is time to ring the self-advocacy bell and let the world know that something is not right here. Sometimes, the smallest things can spur a person into being more aware of self-advocacy, and motivate that person to spend time raising awareness of the autism and Asperger's community.

This is the story of just such an awakening of one young woman, reprinted with permission.

Awakening to Self-Advocacy

"It was just another day, like all days. It was my junior year of college, about six months or so after I had found out I had Asperger's. I hadn't said much about it to anyone because I found no reason to. I didn't know if it was the kind of thing people would be receptive to hearing about. I was still trying to figure out for myself what it all meant. But that all changed one day after an incident in my college library.

I was feeling really groggy that day. Just out of it, a bit overwhelmed, like I couldn't wake up and couldn't focus. I was being over stimulated by the smallest of things. People's voices, people walking around. I needed a break from my work before I could get anything done. I went into the basement bathroom of my college library; the one that hardly anyone ever used, so it assured the most privacy. I went into a stall, locked it and just let my mind run loose with all the thoughts and feelings running through it. Some of them, I said aloud. There was no one else in the bathroom, and there usually wasn't. If someone came in, I would stop talking immediately; but this kind of self-dialogue was a big stress reliever for me.

Thoughts would come and go so fast and be so overwhelming; they were pushing at my brain to get out and couldn't be quieted until I said them out loud, or tried to reason out some of the problems I was struggling with out loud. So, sometimes when I needed to work something out in my head, I would come here for a few minutes to do so, and get a clearer head so I could return to whatever task I had been doing. I realized it sounded weird to talk to yourself, but it was a very accepting atmosphere at my college, and people usually let people alone and didn't judge them. It didn't hurt anyone else to do it, and I stopped when people got nearby. It's just one of many coping mechanisms that adults with Asperger's use to better navigate and cope with their world.

But this particular morning was different. I heard someone come in the bathroom, and stopped talking out loud. Several minutes later, perhaps ten, I heard the door open again and a woman's voice asked me if I was okay. Used to the question, I said "Yeah, I'm fine, just a little bit overwhelmed, I'll be fine," and expected it to end at that, as it usually did. Instead, I got a "Are you sure?" and then the next voice I heard was that of my college security officer asking me to come out. I did so and gasped as I realized college security had filled the bathroom.

"Why were you in there so long?" they asked.

"I....was just trying to calm myself down, you know, just taking a break." I hesitated for a minute, trying to decide whether to say the next part. "I have Asperger's syndrome, and one of the symptoms is severe sensory issues and overload. If I take a few minutes for a time out, then I feel better."

The woman who had started this said, "I'm a psychiatric student at John's Hopkins, about to get my degree. She can't have Asperger's, because she can talk. Asperger's is like autism, and she couldn't talk if she had autism."

I tried to convince her she was mistaken and that Asperger's was very different from what she might have learned about autism. That people with Asperger's certainly could talk, and did so quite well. In response, she threw around a bunch of loaded psychiatric terms about emotional instability that obviously impressed and scared the college cops. They wouldn't listen to me.

"All right, we need to take you to the office and figure out what to do with you," they said.

"What? I'm supposed to meet someone in five minutes. I have work to do."

"No, you need to come with us."

170

They took me to a cavernous, gloomy office in the basement of the library I had never been to, and questioned me for an hour about my behavior and what Asperger's was. I was shaking and so overwhelmed I could barely talk, but I managed to defend myself. Nothing I said made any difference to them. Over my head, they talked about sending me to a hospital, about calling paramedics. They even called in a member of the Baltimore City police, for reasons I will never understand. I wasn't yelling or threatening anyone or myself; I had simply been talking. They tried to call people I knew to confirm what I had said but weren't getting anyone. I kept trying to convince them that I was fine, but they would have none of it. I was desperate to keep them from taking control over me, God Forbid sending me to a hospital when I was just trying to get my sociology homework done. After about an hour of this, one of them finally said, "You know, she really does seem fine now. She seems much better." I internally rolled my eyes and asked if I could please go then. They finally consented. Shaken, I left and made my way back to my dorm room to process everything that had happened to me. I met a friend, the one I was supposed to meet two hours ago, and told her everything that had happened. She was appalled.

I eventually got several heart-felt apologies from both the Residence Life and Security offices on campus. I never did get one from the ignorant John's Hopkins woman who had started the whole thing, and often wished I could write her a letter.

It got me thinking, and gave me a desire to communicate to the world the experience of Asperger's.

I wanted to lay it down unequivocally—this is what an adult with Asperger's looks like. This is what the world looks like to us. Please be aware we may have different needs than you; please do not be alarmed if we present behavior that is unfamiliar to you. Please respect us for who we are, for we have many strengths and positive traits to go along with the things we have difficulty with. Thus motivated, I wrote an editorial about what Asperger's was, and sent it to the Baltimore Sun. I was stunned a few days later to get a phone call informing me that they wanted to publish my article. The article ran on Thanksgiving Day, and I got more than two dozen email replies to it; people telling me they saw their son, daughter, friend, or loved one in what I wrote. People thanking me for describing them so well. I was stunned by the response, and so happy about it. I felt validated and wonderful that I was able to make a difference. After this, I was hooked on self-advocacy. I was invited to speak at two autism conferences in the Northeast as a result of the article. I had essays published in national autism magazines. I had found my voice; a voice that allowed me to educate the world on what being an adult with Asperger's was like. A voice that gave me a sense of meaningfulness and purpose.

So, am I grateful, in a twisted sort of way, for that John's Hopkins student I encountered on that fateful day? Well, I shudder to think of the fate of the people she has treated, and wish I could talk to her personally. But who knows—maybe she has read one of my articles. If it wasn't for her, I'd never be doing what I love, and so maybe it was a good thing after all."

We can see from this essay how important it is to be able to advocate for yourself when you find yourself in uncomfortable situations. If someone if doing something to you that makes you feel uncomfortable, if there are misunderstandings related to AS, you need to be able to communicate for yourself about how to solve them. You need to be able to speak your needs in order to live effectively and safely in the world.

Final Thoughts

In this chapter, we have talked about many different issues. We have discussed the neurodiversity movement, and what the term self-advocacy means. Self-advocacy can mean several different things, from taking political action to change the way adults with Asperger's are perceived nationally, to being able to assert your needs as a person with Asperger's at home, work, or any other environment. Being able to be at least somewhat comfortable in your diagnosis of Asperger's syndrome, knowing when to bring it up and when not to, and knowing how to advocate for yourself are all things that will help you a lot in your daily life.

Joe's Story

Hi My Name is Joe. I was diagnosed with Asperger's when I was 2 years old. As a child I was shy a lot. I liked to be by myself and pretend I was different people like a teacher. My parents tried to get me socially involved by signing me up for t-ball but that did not work out so well. I just sat on the grass and picked it and drew in the dirt.

All through elementary school I had a personal aide to assist me with schoolwork. In 7th and 8th Grade I was put in an Autistic support classroom and mainstreamed for three or four of my classes. 8th Grade was a very tough part of my life. I had foot surgery to correct high arches and was in casts with metal pins in my feet. I still have those metal pins today in a cup as a souvenir. 8th Grade was also a tough year for me not just physically with my foot surgery but mentally and behaviorally as I was always causing trouble. I would not listen to my Mom. I would get into arguments with her yell at her and hit her. Sometimes I got so mad that I took it out on my sister and much to my shame I would hit her also. It got so bad that the police came a couple times and took me to a psychiatric hospital about 3 times over a certain period of time.

Then it got to the point the summer before my freshman year of high school that my parents made the decision to put me in an RTF (Residential Treatment Facility). At first I was not too happy about going there but when I got there they showed me ways to get along better with people. Now six years after that experience at the RTF I look back on it now and think that experience at the RTF really helped me become a better person. I was in an RTF all during my freshman year of high school. I was in the RTF from July 2003 till February 2004. I was released from the RTF in February of 2004 and went to a school that deals with kids who have mental health problems and are not ready to be in the regular public school.

When I first went to that school I was so mad that I couldn't go back to my public school. Someone at that school, I believe it was the therapist at that school, said I would have to earn my way back to my public school. Once I accepted that I was there I worked and was on my best behavior. Finally when the end of the 2004-2005 school years came, my therapist and I sat down to talk about going back to public school. When my therapist said yes I could go back I was so happy. I went back and spent my Junior and senior years of high school at my public school. I graduated from high school in 2007 with honors.

Right now I live with my dad and am going to community college majoring in Graphic Design and I made the dean's list for the fall 2009 semester. I plan to be finished with my associate's degree in December of this year then go look for a job or go on for my bachelor's degree.

I have always had an Interest in one subject or thing. When I was six I was into school buses and outer space.

Then when I got to third grade I started to be interested in the Titanic because I had learned about it. Now my interest is sports. Sometimes this was a benefit because I had something to call my own sometimes it was a distraction because other kids might not be interested in the same things I was.

Aspergers has made it difficult for me to remember things so I use lists. Just recently I was taught how to use the washer and dryer and since I could not remember all the steps like what temperature to wash what clothes in and what settings to put the washer and dryer on. I wrote them down as I was being told them so now I have a visual reminder of what to do. In College I had to learn how to be a self advocate for my needs which I believe is an important thing for adults with mental disabilities to know how to do. Also in college I had accommodations to assist me in my classes like being able to record lectures, extended time on tests and testing outside of the classroom. These accommodations helped me in my classes especially recording my classes. This enabled me to go back and listen to the lecture and take notes at my own pace. Now that some time has passed and my sister and I are getting older our relationship has begun to get better. When I was home from college recently she always came up to me and gave me hugs. For this I was very thankful for. I think the wounds that I caused are beginning to heal.

***

Charlotte's Story

I am a woman who at 27 years old, found out I have Aspergers Syndrome. I would honestly say that I would not wish Aspergers Syndrome on my worst enemy. Due to having Aspergers Syndrome, I have struggled through every aspect of life.

I was told my whole life that I was smart, but I was not measuring up to my potential. I could see some potential now, but I did not see it then. My parents had no idea that I had Aspergers Syndrome. I was expected to achieve the things normal people achieved, but I had to work harder to do those things with no guidance. I was articulate when expressing myself verbally. I could tell people what I had read. Some of what I read was rather mature for me to understand at the age I was at. I did not make it easy for my parents to see that I had a disability. I felt sad because I often disappointed my parents. My mom after finding out I had Aspergers Syndrome was finally proud of me for what I did accomplish, having gotten a new perspective.

I struggled through school. I had to repeat kindergarten because my hand-eye coordination skills were weak. I had to be in a special education class for a time for reading. I did eventually get good at reading and was taken out of the special education class. I had to take three classes over again to be able to graduate from high school, they were Algebra, Biology, and Economics. The first time I took the classes, I did not do very well, but the second time, I earned B's in all three classes. I was late graduating from high school. I finished high school in summer school. I was not the trouble making type, but at times, I really did not pay attention. I was journaling frequently during classes. If I did not like a subject, I would not even bother with it. If I did like a subject, it was an obsession. I hated math, and I loved band and Psychology. I did well in band and psychology.

I knew that I was different from anyone else in my family when I seemed to have sensitivities to everything. I was feeling others pain, physical and emotional. I was even able to know where they were hurting before they said anything about it. In some ways that was hard, having to discern what was mine and what was not, and then not knowing how to deal with it. At other times, I knew what to do and it made it easier for me to help others. It was a lot to deal with feeling my pain and others though. The worst is feeling others anxiety.

I could not stand it as a kid when it was the fourth of July and fireworks were set off. The loud bang scared me. I would cover my ears. Sensitivity to sight and sound is a trigger for migraine headaches I get, which are frequent. Thankfully, I did find some nutritional information that helps with that.

Aspergers Syndrome really had a huge impact on my ability to pick people to date. I was not good at seeing the consequences of what would happen if I dated the wrong guys to be with. My son's biological father had the worst impact on me of any I dated. He was an alcoholic, abandoned his kids, and lied to me about his marital status. I had a guy in front of me who loved me all along, he was there while I was hung up on Mr. Wrong. He was my friend, and there for me as much as possible. Mr. Right rescued me when I was in a homeless shelter and 5 and a half months pregnant. I had decided not to go see Mr. Wrong a few days before I was rescued. I was not dating anyone for 5 months before I decided to date my hero. In that time I read a book called *How to Spot a Dangerous Man*, By Sandra Brown. The book talked about 8 types of Dangerous men, and the women they target. The book was an eye opener for me. The book also talked about how women ignore their red flags that they get about men. I wrote a list of traits I needed a guy to have for me to be willing to date him. I also worked on improving my self esteem. My self esteem had been pretty messed up from having been homeless and pregnant, and from being used by Mr. Wrong. Mr. Wrong has never made an effort to be a dad to our son.

I had issues with keeping jobs. I could not remember verbal instructions. I once had a boss ask me "are you stupid or something?" I really did not have the emotional means at the time to handle that. I was going to be homeless the next day and I was pregnant, so being emotional would have been easy anyway. I also was not getting enough hours at that job. I quit that job. At another job I had, I was doing fine washing dishes, up until I burnt my arm in the 200 degree sanitation water. That was one painful experience. I could have gone back to that job, but in that case, I was scared of hot water after that. I was accident prone, I guess issues with motor skills still plague me. Ironically, I am a great dancer.

Parenting has probably been the toughest part of having Aspergers Syndrome. My husband was on a ship working for four months at a time. I was alone a chunk of the time taking care of my son. I had a poor time of it trying to remember important things I had to do, like arranging doctor's appointments. I had trouble getting organized, so I wasted time, which I only had a limited amount of time. I got overwhelmed easily, and my son needed plenty of attention so that was not a good thing. I would get irritated when I got overwhelmed and that happened fast.

I wanted so much to be a good mom, but motherhood has been a nightmare, having this. I read parenting material to try to be a better mom, but then the information does not stick when I try to apply it. I had to read information on parenting and then apply it immediately, or it does not get done. I took parenting classes. I had to figure out what my son needed by process of elimination because I could not read his cues when he was younger. My son was taken out of my home 3 times, the 3rd time being over a pacifier

178

that was around his neck. My son had a seizure and the pacifier got tight around his neck. I am still fighting for him. I have avoided putting anything around my son's neck since then. My self esteem has been impacted severely by this and my heart broken. I love my son, but motherhood has not been something that has come naturally to me. My son suffers because of my failings as a mom. My son has been in foster care, and he is with loved ones now, but he goes between 3 places. I think it gets confusing for my boy.

I know it is good for me to have pride in who I am but for me, if I could get rid of the negative parts that interfere with my ability to lead a happy and fulfilling life, I would do it. I want a better life for myself and for my son too. I am looking up as much information as I can find about every possible thing that can cause Aspergers symptoms, from metal toxicity, vaccines, to nutritional components, and leaky gut syndrome, and digestional problems, and how the mind works. Thankfully, I seem to find health and psychology riveting and love to study them. I think there is hope for me and all of those people who have Aspergers Syndrome. I am glad I found out I have Aspergers Syndrome, because now I have the power to make changes. My advice to parents of children with Asperger's Syndrome, and those with Asperger's Syndrome is do not give up on finding solutions. Your child or you can have a better life than the one I have led.

Charlotte

***

8. How to Lead a Meaningful Life: Depression and Meaning in Your Life

Well, at this point we have covered friends, relationships, employment and social services. For those with AS, you know how to at least start making friends, how to go after the opposite sex, and how to start to have all the trappings of what most people would consider a decent life. But what if it still isn't enough?

You have a place to live, you have a source of income, you're trying to do the whole living independently thing and by all accounts succeeding. Someone from the outside might look in and think you have a pretty good life. Hey, you go to work at 9, you put in eight hours, you get a paycheck, and you support yourself. That alone is pretty good. But, sometimes it is not enough. Sometimes, life can feel pretty empty even when you are doing what you think you should be doing. Sometimes it can feel devoid of meaning. Maybe you haven't even gotten that far. Maybe you don't yet have a job or maybe you never will. Maybe you're even living at your parents' house and unable to get out and live on your own. Again, how do you find meaning in your life? How do you want to get up in the morning, how can you make life matter to you?

In this chapter, we will discuss the issues of making life meaningful for adults with Asperger's.

The Issue—Difficulty Accessing The World

Anyone can tell you that life is more than a paycheck, more than just a mere existence. You don't have to have Asperger's to realize that. People all over the world suffer from depression and boredom about their lives. But for people who have Asperger's, it can be even more difficult. Accessing the world and participating in all of the daily rituals—that so many people without AS do without even thinking about it—can be much more difficult for an adult with AS.

Just a few examples

1. Friends

All the friends that often come easily, or at least more easily, for typical people are a huge struggle for people with AS. They do not make friends easily. This means loneliness, isolation, lack of someone to go to the movies with, a concert with, or out to dinner with. Lack of needed support, lack of help for things around the house or personal support or other needs only a friend can fill.

2. Difficulty accessing public facilities due to sensory issues

Restaurants may be too loud, a beach too crowded, movie theaters too loud, shops too smelly. Sensory issues can interfere a lot with someone with AS going out and having a good time. Nightclubs, bars, a number of places are usually too loud for those with AS. Any place with too much going on at once is usually out. This makes finding things to do with a friend challenging even if the person with AS has managed to find one.

3. Easily overwhelmed

Trying to read faces, trying to read social cues, trying to multitask, filtering sensory information—all the things a person with AS has to go through in a typical day can make them exhausted! Even a short time in public interacting with others can be more than those with AS can sometimes handle. Workplace politics, noisy people on a bus, unexpected schedule changes, bad weather, all kinds of things can bring a person with AS to the brink of being overwhelmed pretty quickly. And once they are overwhelmed, they stop functioning pretty quickly. There is only so much you can handle until you just have to stop. This, again, makes the world less accessible and makes it harder to participate in the world in ways that make you feel good.

4. Trouble with office politics

A lot of people make friends easily in the office, and automatically get invited to office parties, sporting events, get-togethers and so on. Someone with AS who sticks out in the office, doesn't make small talk or chit chat, and doesn't seem friendly and inviting on the outside may get left out, and this can be depressing for someone who wants to be involved.

5. Clothing

Some people with AS have difficulty wearing clothing that looks "hip" or even appropriate due to severe sensory issues. They may prefer all cotton to jeans, and hate anything that involves dressing up. If you can't dress the part, it is often harder to be taken seriously by the circles of the world you want to be a part of. Some people with AS could wear the "right" clothes but just simply do not know what to wear.

So, you may have the job and the apartment, or you may not, but either way you have problems filling time in a way that is meaningful to you. Sure, you have your hobbies, and they are fulfilling, but once in a while you want to grab a dinner with a buddy or not go to the movies alone; you want to not be the one person who is standing at the edge of a conversation about a weekend activity and be the only one NOT invited. You want to feel like you matter to someone.

The Spoon Theory: Considerations for Adults with Asperger's in Interacting with the World

One way to understand the trouble that adults with Asperger's often have in accessing the world is to use the analogy of the Spoon Theory. This is a great essay that Christine Miserandino of ButYouDontLookSick.com wrote in 2003. Christine's website deals with invisible illnesses and the effects that they can have on those who have them. Asperger's is in many ways an invisible illness, because those who have it don't LOOK sick or disabled, they look perfectly normal, like any other adult. But then when they open their mouths, they are likely to engage in some kind of social gaffe or come off in the wrong way.

They are thought of as stupid or as having character flaws rather than as just lacking in social knowledge. Adults with AS can get overwhelmed and have a meltdown—yes, even adults still have meltdowns, to different degrees—and people think they're just being stubborn, or self-centered, or have serious emotional problems, when they're simply just overwhelmed and need some time to themselves. People with AS can be judged as lazy when they don't perform all the tasks their peers do at the same speed as their peers. Few realize how much effort that many daily tasks take adults with AS due to anxiety, sensory issues, processing issues, or lack of social knowledge.

The spoon theory posits that you only have a limited store of energy per day and you have to be thinking all the time to plan how to use it wisely. In effect, you only have a certain number of "spoons."

Christine, who has an illness that causes a lot of fatigue called lupus, tried to explain it to a friend of hers like this:

"Most people start the day with unlimited amounts of possibilities, and energy to do whatever they desire, especially young people. For the most part, they do not need to worry about the effects of their actions. So for my explanation, I used spoons to convey this point. I wanted something for her to actually hold, for me to then take away, since most people who get sick feel a "loss" of a life they once knew. If I was in control of taking away the spoons, then she would know what it feels like to have someone or something else, in this case Lupus, being in control. I asked her to list off the tasks of her day, including the most simple. As she rattled off daily chores, or just fun things to do, I explained how each one would cost her a spoon.

It's hard, the hardest thing I ever had to learn is to slow down, and not do everything. I fight this to this day. I hate feeling left out, having to choose to stay home, or to not get things done that I want to. I wanted her to feel that frustration. I wanted her to understand, that everything everyone else does comes so easy, but for me it is one hundred little jobs in one. I need to think about the weather, my temperature that day, and the whole day's plans before I can attack any one given thing. When other people can simply do things, I have to attack it and make a plan like I am strategizing a war. It is in that lifestyle, the difference between being sick and healthy. It is the beautiful ability to not think and just do. I miss that freedom. I miss never having to count "spoons".

I think it isn't just good for understanding Lupus, but anyone dealing with any disability or illness. Hopefully, they don't take so much for granted or their life in general. I give a piece of myself, in every sense of the word when I do anything. It has become an inside joke. I have become famous for saying to people jokingly that they should feel special when I spend time with them, because they have one of my 'spoons.'"

Christine might have been writing this about a physical disability, but as she says in the end, it really can be applied to many other disabilities as well. Adults with Asperger's often get frustrated because they need to plan out their days and time, often to the minute, in order to feel at all comfortable and functional. They often cannot engage in spur of the moment activities. They often can't join in noisy, boisterous activities their peers are participating in because it's just too overwhelming. Often times going out of the house at all can be a big gamble. They have to decide if the toll the sensory aspects of going out will take on them is worth it. They are in a sense strategizing as if in a war. Can I handle this? Is it worth it? Will I get overloaded? Will I have a meltdown? Can I put on the "social face" I need to? In this sense, then, when someone gets one of their "spoons"—when an adult with AS decides to engage in an activity—those they are participating with should feel very lucky indeed. Again, the limited amount of social and emotional energy an adult with AS has for interacting with the outside world can be very frustrating to them (and those around them) and can contribute to feelings of anxiety and depression when the adult wants to be able to participate more.

Depression and Anxiety in Adults with Asperger's

Depression and anxiety can be huge problems in adults with Asperger's. When they get older and realize that they still have more limitations than they would like, this can be hugely frustrating. Adults with Asperger's have very

185

variable strengths and difficulties. Some can hold down jobs, some can't. Some have friends, some don't. Some can live on their own and some can't. When you get older, more awareness comes. The younger child or teenager may not have realized how different they were from everyone else, but the adult usually does.

The 40 year old who is making $75,000 a year as an accountant may seem successful, but on the inside is very critical of himself for never being able to get a girl or have a conversation that lasts for longer than three minutes with any of his co-workers. The 30 year old who never managed to leave home blames himself every day for living at his parents' and not having a job. The 60 year old who has worked all her life and tried to give back to the world as best she could feels depressed because she never managed to make any lasting connections in her life. It goes on and on.

Anxiety can be a huge problem with adults with AS. They have a lot of living skills but they still don't know how to perform socially a lot of the time. They still struggle with what to say, what words to use, tone of voice, body language. They fear rejection and they are used to it. They know that they are not received well by others but have no idea what to do about it.

They are tired of being the odd one out. In the coffee break room, in the grocery store, at the church picnic. The small talk does not come easily. Fear of messing up, fear of being judged, can cause a lot of anxiety. Many adults simply do not want to try anymore. Sometimes, anxiety can hurt a person's job because it's too difficult to talk and perform social functions at work. Sometimes, it will cripple the person and make them afraid to leave their house.

Depression comes hand in hand with this. If you don't feel your life is meaningful, then it is very, very easy to become depressed. Adults with Asperger's often feel their life has no purpose. Indeed, sometimes it doesn't. Because of tantrums, meltdowns, and sensory problems, a lot of adults with Asperger's are not able to leave home and participate in the world in any meaningful way.

These are usually very intelligent people, often with college degrees or higher, who can work their way around a classroom or textbook but not around people in the real world, not around a workplace and its office politics.

Many adults resent living at their parents' house still, and rightfully so. Some adults compare themselves to their more social, gregarious peers and fall short. Many just feel there is no reason to get up in the morning. They are trying to mold themselves to a world that just doesn't fit them. Even the successful ones feel a void of meaning because they are not doing things that matter to them. So many adults have skills and intelligence but no way to use it.

An August 2009 article in the Times newspaper out of London, entitled "How do autistic children survive in adults?", portrays this challenge very articulately.

"Peter Griffin is 29, he has an IQ of 159, a degree in astrophysics, and a gallows humour about his Asperger's syndrome, an autistic-spectrum disorder that makes social interaction so difficult that his longest—indeed his only—stretch of paid work has been a Saturday job in Tesco, which he has had since he was 16. He is so wired after his shift that he is awake until 4 am and it takes him the rest of the week to recover: "At the end of a day trying to be 'normal', acting the part, wearing the mask and reining myself in, I'm like a pressure cooker."

Peter is smart but doesn't have the practical skills to fit into the world. Sometimes with support, adults with Asperger's can find positions and jobs that match their skills, but it usually takes support from organizations that have limited funds and ability to help. There is a need for more support for adults with AS to interact with and work in the world.

"Ann has explored the idea of Peter working as a teaching assistant. He did an eight-week programme with a council-run scheme called Work Solutions. "He was very, very motivated. They said, 'We'll allocate someone to work with you in a few weeks.'" But three months went by and nobody phoned. Peter's mood plummeted. His conclusion was: "I don't know anything is happening, so I'll assume nothing is happening.""

Robyn, a 22 year old with Asperger's also featured in the same article, talks about how hard it can be to be with people:

"It's like you have a jar in your head and you have emotional tokens which swoosh round, so you've got a constant flow. With people on the autistic spectrum, the jar gets full really, really quickly and then it explodes and they get scared and they don't know what to do."

Robyn found a way to have meaningful activity in her life, though, through support programs and networking with local organizations:

"Robyn's experiences at school were so bad, she says, that "I thought I'd be a homeless drug addict by the time I was 21." She was sent to social-skills classes: "Ate biscuits—pretty useless really." But at college, thanks to a proper transition and good learning support, everything went right.

She is now a self-employed mentor for Aspie children, with referrals coming from SENCOs (special-needs coordinators) and parents."

Autistic Kids Turn Into Autistic Adults

Autistic kids turn into autistic adults, a reality that many in the world have not yet realized. Most supports end at age 18 or 21. There is often no help for aging parents who have to manage kids-turned adults, the once cute 10 year old who is now 20 or 30 and still has meltdowns, still has a limited understanding of the world and how it works, and still has nowhere to go.

Many adults with Asperger's sit in their parents' basements all day because they have nowhere to go. While there are some job training programs and organizations to support adults with Asperger's, they are few and far between, can be hard to get into, and vary in quality. There simply need to be more organizations that teach adults with Asperger's basic living skills, job employment skills, and living in the world skills, as well as provide respite to parents who can't handle all the care needed.

Amy Brosnan's parents know only too well the first hand reality the lack of services for adults with ASD causes.

"Amy Brosnan, an ethereal 19-year-old lodged somewhere between childhood and adulthood, was diagnosed with autism at 11. There was a lot of "holding down" at her first school, which Amy remembers as "all fear and no learning". Since she turned 12, she has been at home; she has had no suitable education at all. And now, her mother, Cathy, believes, she has no future."

It can all be summed up by Rosie Cousins' quote about her drug addicted adult son with Asperger's. "I love him dearly," she writes. "I don't want his life's journey to be a worthless one."

Indeed. No one wants their child to live a worthless life. No person wants their life to be worthless. But unfortunately, with all the barriers to life and participation that those with AS face, it can often feel that this is exactly the case.

The Search for Meaning in Adults with AS

Depression and feelings of meaninglessness in life is a common discussion topic of adults with Asperger's. There is much discussion of it to be found on Internet discussion groups, such as Wrongplanet.net, an online community for people with Asperger's.

In a discussion about feeling sad and lonely, user Mosto talks about the lack of meaningful human contact in his life.

"I drove 40 km yesterday to buy a chair and run errands. I was so sad inside. But didn't let on. My mum says she doesn't understand. No contact with human being except paying for items."

User Funaho talked about feeling hopeless in the mornings and having trouble getting himself up for the day, a sentiment a lot of adults with Asperger's often feel.

"I know how you feel, though for me it's usually mornings that are bad. I get what a lot of people seem to call "morning dread" where I just wake up feeling completely hopeless and alone, and often times I have to argue with myself just to get up and go to work."

Finally, user ActivebutOdd talks about feeling depressed about things she could not do but others could.

"I get that too. The internet is a good distraction, but it has pitfalls. Like when other people's activities come up and they're enjoying things you can't do. Anyway, rambling. I feel for you Fickle."

190

Some people go on medication to help with feelings of depression and anxiety. Antidepressants, such as Prozac and Zoloft, can often be helpful in lifting the depressive feeling. Sometimes, anti anxiety meds can be helpful at resolving feelings of anxiety. Therapy and support groups can often help with feelings of depression and feelings of meaninglessness. These are very real feelings and they need to be addressed one way or another. Talking about them and getting support from another person is very important. Your doctor will be able to give you referrals to psychiatrists or therapists that can help.

Glad to be Different's Story

I am 39 and I believe I grew up without a diagnosis. I was the first person in kindergarten to learn to read, I could memorize very well. But I got laughed at for not being able to draw a circle even after the teacher showed me. In first grade, I was taken out of my class and sent to the 2nd grade class during reading time because I was advanced. This upset me because I was not with my friends and I was plunged into a new social group that I didn't understand or wasn't familiar with. So I corrected this by hating reading and it solved my problem as a kid. I didn't get taken out of my class again.

In elementary school, I learned very quickly from the girls who were in gymnastics the moves they were doing on the bar and enjoyed it very much. I wished I could be in it too. Until my uncle saw my skill and over praised me on it. He said that I WOULD be in the Olympics, totally bypassing my choice in the matter, so I made up my mind right then and there that he would be wrong, and I never did it again. I have been called perfectionist, preacher by my peers in a way that made me feel on the outside of the group, stubborn, and I hate change big time!

In Jr. High and High School, I didn't do very well socially as I would have liked to. I have always felt like I was on the outside of the group looking in. Church allowed me to find something that I was good at and showed me that it is okay to be different. So I put my effort to excel into church during that time and it got me through beautifully. I too am happy with the way I am, but I know that I do things, like, the way I dress, that cause people to look at me quizzically and humorously.

I don't like to wear uncomfortable clothes, I don't care how cute they are. I have learned to laugh at myself too and believe that it is a gift, especially when I see how disturbed some people get over perfectly fitting in. I just don't care anymore. It doesn't seem to be a problem in college, in fact they encourage "individuals" at that age. So it worked for me. I encourage my son, who has been diagnosed with Asperger's Syndrome, that in college he will fit in better and that someday if he keeps his chin up, he may be the boss of the losers that have been bullying him. It's just 6-7 years of your life and then it gets better, I tell him.

All of my life, I am interested in psychology and what makes people tick. Why do they do the things that they do. They are so different than me. But the more I look the more I realize, that they are not so different. They are just controlled more by what others think of them. Okay, maybe I'm not witty and there are jokes that will fly over my head, but I like who I am, I have friends who seem to need my strength of hope through difficult times. I do believe it is a gift! I think it runs in my family. My mom won't hear of it though which is fine. But I think she has it big time as she has never been able to keep friends on an intimate level as she has wanted to. Like me, they come and seek out her spiritual advice and admire her from a safe distance. Yeah, she can make you feel uncomfortable when she doesn't think you are doing something right.

I saw her grief growing up when she struggled to fit in. I saw her in a dark living room crying and sometimes when I was older picking my brain on how she could make and keep friends better. She thought that if you invited people over to your house that they would invite you to theirs and you would be friends. We had over half of the county come through our doors last we counted. She was well known for her hospitality and social awkwardness. But I love her and admire her bravery. She never gives up trying.

She gave up on regular people and went to the streets to take care of the homeless. She was scared of them at first but knows them each by name now and cares for them like a bossy mom. She's not afraid to correct the mother who uses her girl to beg. She will give her a verbal reprimand right there in public. I have seen that it takes someone like my mom to be able to ignore social standards in order to bring about change and think outside the box.

Many people in different churches and organizations have come alongside of her and a grassroots kind of thing has sprung up. She is brilliant on problem solving skills and still adds to her education, though she didn't do very well in school. Even in her older age, she has memorized large chapters of the Bible.

I am watching my daughter who is 8 years old. I have seen some genius in her and I have seen some similar struggles socially. I may have enough evidence to get her diagnosed early, before the social stigma of a label will mean much.

Well, I don't usually share on these things, but if there is a way that you can use it to help other girls who may have similar struggles as we have had, then please do so.

Sincerely,

Ms. Glad to Be Different

***

How to Lead a Meaningful Life

The most important thing to help change these feelings of depression and meaninglessness is to figure out how to lead a meaningful life! I know, I know, easier said than done, right? Therapy is great and can help, but the BIGGEST thing you can do for yourself is to figure out how to change your life so you actually enjoy it. Figure out what you can do that will add a little oomph to your life, a little spice. Do something beyond just the usual 9-5 work routine. Do something different. Join a club. Go out to lunch with someone you've never talked to before. Start volunteering somewhere. If you live at home and don't go out much, figure out ways to broaden your horizons. The following are several ways you can find meaning in your life.

1. Volunteer somewhere

Volunteering is one of the most important things you can do to raise your self esteem and get you feeling good about the world. It makes you feel a part of things, it makes you feel connected. Giving back to the world makes you feel like you have value. There are many, many different ways you can volunteer somewhere. Think about what your interests are.

- Do you like working with kids? Volunteer at an after school program or daycare program. Mentor a younger kid.

- Tutor someone in a subject you know a lot about.

- Do you like to write? Volunteer to write for a local newsletter, write a blog, or submit letters to the editor or editorials to the local newspaper.

- Spend a day at a soup kitchen, if the noise is not an issue for you. Volunteer for Meals on Wheels.

- Visit the elderly.

- Volunteer for a clean-up day at a local park or river.

- Do some clerical work for a local nonprofit.

- Don't want to be around people much but still want something to do? Volunteer at the local library, straightening books on the shelves or going through new or returned inventory.

- If you like animals, volunteer at an animal shelter.

- If you like to garden, offer your services to an elderly person who needs help.

There are many opportunities, many different things you can do.

If you need help finding opportunities in your area, go to the website www.volunteermatch.com, and type in your zip code. You will see many different opportunities pop up. The nice thing about volunteering is that people WANT you to be there, and they are often more forgiving if you are a bit socially awkward because you are providing a good service to them.

2. Document the world

If you like to take pictures, get a camera and start documenting your world. Publish the pictures online.

3. Take up a hobby

Hobbies are one of the best ways to combat loneliness and depression. Find something that gives you joy.

4. Learn how to cook

Eating can be a great way to feel better, when done in moderation of course, and the satisfaction of knowing you created what you are eating can be immense.

5. Reading

Take up reading—reading can be a great way to explore other worlds.

6. Exercise

Get into exercising—exercising is a good way to keep away depression. Start walking, biking, jogging. Go to the local pool and swim. Join a sports team. There are many groups that you can join that are associated with exercise. It is easy to join a fitness club with regularly scheduled classes. Many times it is easier to chat with people before and after doing something physical because you have some specific shared event to discuss.

7. Join a social group

Find an area related to your interests. Chess, writing, photography, whatever. Join a local Asperger's group. Find a drop in center for people with disabilities.

The important thing is to work around your limitations as best as possible. Think about what you want most out of life. Then think about what is keeping you from it. As best as possible try to think of ways around the obstacles. If you can only work from home, try to find a writing job or something using the phone. If you don't want to be around people, find a job or volunteer opportunity that doesn't require you to be. If you can't work for long stretches of time, find a place that will let you come in for only a couple of hours. **You have to make the most out of your life, and you have to take the initiative to find things to do with it that are enjoyable to you**. Once you get involved with something—anything!—you will almost definitely start to feel better about your life.

What if the Aspie adult in my life refuses to help himself?

One of the most common questions that parents or other people with loved ones who have Asperger's ask is "How can I get help for my son/daughter etc. who does not want to be helped?"

That is a tough one, of course. Once the person with AS is an adult, they can pretty much do what they want. Especially if they are living on their own, there is very little you can do. Even if they are still living with you, as is often the case, it may seem as if all they want to do is stay in their room and play on the computer. So how do you motivate them to get help?

Unfortunately, most likely you can't. Someone who doesn't want help will be very resistant to it. But you can give them encouragement. Give them consistent and gentle messages. Say things like, "I can see you are lonely and frustrated. How about joining a chess group? You love to play chess, and this way you make friends with others and do something you love. How about you go once and if you don't like it, you don't have to go back?" Offer to drive them if they don't drive. Leave literature about different clubs, groups or other programs that could help lying around for them to peruse. Try to get them to see why it could be valuable to them and assuage any fears they might have. Tell them people won't judge them (if that seems like it would be the case), have them talk to people you know who have also gone to whatever program you are trying to encourage. If you think they can be bribed, you might also try that, although it can have varying results. Perhaps with some extra money or some item they've wanted to buy. Perhaps with a trip somewhere they like.

If it's therapy you're trying to encourage, the same approach can be used. Try to understand the reason the adult has for not engaging in the activity and how they can be resolved. Find activities with only a limited amount of contact with other people, or a therapist that seems like they will be especially attuned to what your loved one needs. The most important thing is to be there for your loved one, and reassure them that you will always be there for them whatever they choose.

It can be frustrating to stand back and watch but sometimes that is all you can do. If you live with your adult child and they have behaviors you can't tolerate, you can try to get in home care to work with them and take some of the pressure off, or even respite care. You can try to place them into a supported living house. The best way to motivate a person to change is to relate the change to their interests. If all they do is sit at home and play video games, find a video game convention that they can go to and meet people. At least it will be social contact. Then ask them questions about who they met and what they did. It will be a form of connection between the two of you.

Everyone wants to lead a meaningful life. Everyone wants to have a reason to get up in the morning. Adults with Asperger's are no exception. Due to problems they have with interacting and accessing the world in the same manner as everyone else, much depression and anxiety can ensue. Sometimes, an adult with AS can look pretty functional from the outside, but be wondering inside what the point of it all is. Many adults with AS have the skills to be functional in the world but lack the support to be able to do so, so are relegated to meaningless existences.

There are ways to get involved in the world, though, to minimize this depression and lack of meaningful activity. Finding what makes you happy and finding a way to engage in it; that is the task we all have for ourselves, as simple as it sounds. The key to a meaningful life is being able to overcome your difficulties to do what you love, in some shape or form.

Charles' Story

I'm a 59 year old with Asperger's and epilepsy. I'm now retired from a 30 year career in the US Federal Government, so you might say I'm one of the very lucky ones. However, my success came after struggling with something I didn't quite understand until 2008. It took that long to discover I was a member of the greater Asperger's community.

As a child, I remember my mom saying I didn't talk for the longest time and my movements were always kind of clumsy and awkward. She wouldn't let me do normal activities like a little boy would do. She thought me too accident prone and I guess a little bit slower than others.

Socially, I was very shy from my earliest years and I hated any attention drawn to myself. My memories of childhood are still very vivid to this day, and as I've read in your newsletters, I was prone to bullying by other children and adults too. Fortunately, I was a very quiet child, often not acknowledging or responding to the verbal abuse directed at me. Sometimes they just got bored and left me alone after that.

I think the bullying just about stopped when I reached the senior year of high school. By then, I was so quiet and inside myself that I treasured my anonymity. I was kind of proud that I was quiet, never started fights or longed for attention. I had my own little fantasy world and I had very focused interests in cars and history. I also drew a lot and never let on to anyone of my talents. My mom discovered my drawing ability by accident. I would draw secretly and once in a while would post one or two on my bedroom wall. Then she came to me completely surprised, wondering where the talent came from. I'd never wanted to show off, and I was kind of secretive about everything. I guess I didn't trust people with my secret, still I didn't know a thing about Aspergers. This was still back in the dark ages in the late sixties.

I was smart enough to go to college, but it took me ten years and about 3 tries before I got my degree in accounting. I chose accounting because it was very repetitive and it suited my personality. I was also considering art as a career, but art was too personal and close to me so I kept that as my lifelong hobby. Six months after graduating from college in 1979, I was able to land a job with the Federal government in accounting, which I stuck with for 30 years, retiring in 2008.

To backtrack a few years, I met my wife Carolyn in 2003 through a dating service. We married after a quick six month courtship. She was my first and only relationship. I think before she came along I had all of 3 dates that I can remember, all with different women. I was over 30 years old on my first date. So you can see why I was puzzled about life because everything that mattered in my life came hard for me. Except that my understanding and tolerance about people who are different just grew more and more over the years. I always seemed to relate to and felt comfortable with people who were outside the mainstream.

Upon moving to Arizona from the US east coast in June 2008, I followed up with a new neurologist about my epilepsy, which was diagnosed in 1987. MRI technology had advanced enough in 20 years so that my doctor was able to diagnose that I had grey matter heterotopias, which is a brain disorder from before birth. Following that news in 2008, the association to Asperger's was also made. Now I'm retired and happy, knowing that there were good reasons for all that had happened to me during my lifetime. I also realize how blessed I am because I consider having Asperger's to be a blessing. It taught me tolerance and forgiveness. I am not bitter, rather I'm happy knowing.

Charles G.,

Retired Happy Person

***

Anonymous

This is my story:

From my earliest age I felt afraid and lonely; still today I have a deathly fear of heights. Up through my high school years I found it extremely hard to make and keep friends, even though I tried hard; I could not understand why! Especially in my high school years, even though I played sports, played in the band and was very involved in school activities, I was extremely lonely and often cried at night; I would take long walks at night trying to make myself feel better. I survived my childhood through obsessive compulsive involvement in religion. Through adulthood I could not make friends and accepted my lonely fate, but always wondered what was wrong with me?

At about age 40, as my world was crumbling around me, a psychiatrist quickly diagnosed me suffering from severe depression! This "tag" never ever occurred to me. So, for the next fifteen years I tried six different SSRI drugs to cure what was wrong with me, but all of them failed over time to help the depression, the anger, the loneliness inside me. I actually thought at times I must be from "another dimension" or just "crazy"! I did marry and we had four children; the courtship and early years of family were wonderful, but the pressure of raising a family and working difficult jobs started to unravel me mentally.

I was blaming my wife for everything that was wrong and found myself distancing from her. Cancer took my wife from me, and three years after her passing I suddenly realized that the last ten years of our marriage I WAS extremely selfish and only cared about myself! This shocking revelation devastated me and I continued on anti-depressive but felt lost AND more angry. Someone I knew had sudden outbursts of anger; finally, this person went to a specialist and was diagnosed with mild "Asperger's Syndrome".

One time casually I picked up some of the literature he had and I almost FELL OVER DEAD! Just about every symptom I was reading applied exactly to me from my earliest years. For the next many months I read everything on Aspergers including Kendall's book.

I was ecstatic at finally knowing "what was wrong with me" and convinced my therapist I had Aspergers Syndrome. I went off my Effexor but soon realized I would still need to take an anti-depressant for the rest of my life. I also found "religion" again through a Medium, and my life is better (mentally) than it has been for a long time; I've even been able to cut my medicine in half. I got Asperger's either when my mom's heart stopped during my birth or I got the genes from an early mentally ill ancestor!

Please do not use my name.

***

Robby's Story

Hello Craig, call me Robby please.

I've struggled with Aspergers Syndrome my whole life. Since I was a little kid, I had problems socializing with others and reading people. My anger has been extremely out of control and to this day I can never get a hold of it. I ran away several times when I was a kid and drove myself nuts trying to figure out if I was crazy or not.

At my preschool in Kenya, my teachers were amazed that I was so bright and how inquisitive I was, so they got me a 10 volume encyclopedia for my 5th birthday. In first grade, my passion to learn hadn't receded, so my teacher suggested that I be screened. I was diagnosed ADHD with an IQ of 158, but they seemed to miss the Asperger's. I lived in Kenya up until I was 10 years old, in Grade 4. Moving to the USA was probably the hardest transition of my life. The people at my new school picked on me because I was different, and I always felt like an outcast. I was strangely tall for my age, and that didn't help. The social awkwardness and disappointment went on until I was 13.

I read about a condition called "Asperger's Syndrome" in a column in the Washington Post, and started to research it. I was tested and diagnosed that same year. I felt so much better after that, that I had a reason for feeling the way I do, why I like rocking back and forth, not being able to handle my emotions, and so forth.

My social life went on awkwardly, but I knew why that was, so it didn't matter. My life hasn't been limited very much, except for the social interactions. I had a lot of challenge reading people's faces, body language, and with my anger. Many of the boys in middle and high school wanted to beat me up, probably because of faulty logic, that if you can beat up the biggest guy, you must be the king. They picked fights with me and I knocked them out. I saw the headmaster a lot. I passed school with a GPA of 3.94, went to MIT, and I'm now a neurologist, and I study the impact of drugs on the brain. It's my dream job. It took a lot of self control to get past the emotional side of things, but I'm kind of glad that I have Asperger's, it makes me...unique. I have a girlfriend who's also an Aspie, so we understand each other. I hope to marry her and move back to Kenya, or maybe Australia, where my dad is from.

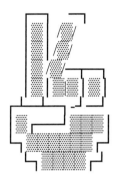

```
(\__/)
(=' '=)
(")_(")
```

***

9. Getting an Asperger's Diagnosis as an Adult

If you are lucky, you got diagnosed with Asperger's when you were a kid, and got the proper treatment to help you cope. You had years to deal with it and come to terms with what being different meant. However, for most adults with Asperger's in the present day and time, that is not the case. Asperger's was not even recognized as an official disorder per the DSM, the official handbook of what is and isn't a disorder, until 1994. Most of today's adults were simply too young at that time to have gotten the proper diagnosis. There was no awareness among doctors. That means many adults grew up with a sense of shame, of always wondering what was wrong with them. They also missed out on treatments that could have helped them better cope with some of the issues that come with Asperger's syndrome. However, it is not too late for adults to get a diagnosis, at any age. There are many reasons to get a diagnosis even as an adult. This chapter will explore how and why to find out if you have Asperger's in your adulthood.

Lone Wolf's Story

My story,

Kids made fun of me in school because I guess they think I was weird. I wasn't diagnosed until I was 17, I'm 19 now.

I always had trouble in school because kids were mean to me and the older I got the worse I was doing on my work because I didn't understand the work, because I didn't ask for help, even though I'm smart. So in 7th grade they sent me to a Special Ed school, which was a school for BD kids, they had behavior problems; I think I was mainly sent there for failing my classes. That school was not good for me, I stayed in Sp Ed school from 7th grade all the way till I graduated high school. I was in two different Sp Ed schools.

In the 8th grade my school sent me to a psych hospital because of the way I was behaving and because I told them something, but they misunderstood what I said, I was there for 8 days. When I was 16 the police came to my school and took me to jail because the teachers aid thought I was trying to stab him with a pencil but I was trying to pull away from him so I could get away, because I was in the room and I was supposed to be doing my work, but I was just having a bad day.

When the police came I was crying and screaming, they put handcuffs on me and said do you want to go to jail. One guy had his knee on the back of my knee and it hurt so bad. They never told me I was under arrest or read me my rights, they drove me right to the jail. I was screaming and crying all the way there. Then when I got there they strapped me to this black chair. I was shaking so bad that they had a hard time strapping me in, then one guy shocked me in the back of the neck with something and the other guy said she's a juvenile, so I don't think they were supposed to do that. They left me there for about an hour I screamed and cried the worst I ever have in my whole life. Then some other guy came and they put me in shackles, hands and feet, then took me to the juvenile jail.

I had never been in trouble with the law or been to jail so I was scared. I won't tell about the details after they took me there, but I was there a month and then all the charges were cleared. But after that I was traumatized. When I went to the new Sp Ed school I never really talked that much or hardly even moved. I didn't want people to notice or pay attention to me. For years in school I always had to listen to cussing and nasty language from the other students.

Then when I was 17 a psychiatrist diagnosed me with Asperger's Syndrome, but a few years earlier my aunt suggested it to my old school but the principal said no way. The psychiatrist only gave me, my mom and my grandma a paper with questions on it. We filled it out, gave it back to her then she diagnosed me. From what I've read, diagnosing Asperger's takes more than one doctor and more time and more information than filling out a paper. So who knows if I was diagnosed right. But I graduated high school and now I am about to start collage, God helped me through it all. With God all things are possible.

Lone Wolf

***

Richard's Story

My name is Richard. I am 19 years old. I've just found out I've got Asperger's. It makes me feel better knowing they've found out what's wrong with me. One of my symptoms is I think people are looking at me and laughing at me. Another one of my symptoms is I feel people look at me because I'm stiff. At school I was bullied for a year. I'm worried about going out. I'm very good at maths and art and I like music.

***

Ray's Story

Aspergers, for me, has been a disability in a few ways. As a youth, Aspergers was not classified in the autism spectrum and so I suffered not knowing what was wrong with me, wanting answers, solutions on how to fix it. My mother was told there may be some level of autism but she refused to accept any kind of possibility that I may be different, "defective" as she would see it, and so, without any sort of counseling or help of any kind, I suffered quietly in my own world.

I couldn't fit in and play with other children, I just couldn't. I didn't know how to fit in, always feeling awkward in a social setting. I always sought the rear of a classroom, watched others on a corner of the playground or played with just one other child. I always had just one good friend, fortunately for me, someone always reached out, always just one other child.

Without any help on how to deal with this syndrome, I started to become bitter with the world and everyone in it, getting into fights when I have had enough humiliation from the other children and feeling the world will never change for me, that I will never fit in. As life went on into adulthood, my torment was less because I just avoided people, lived in my own world with art and photography as a comfort. I excelled and was stimulated by art, especially photography which friends would buy.

Women were attracted to me, but I could never make the first move. The one woman that did show interest, I devoted my time to her, eventually marrying her, and having 2 daughters. Later my art and photography diminished to nothing as I tried to make a living. I was offered a technical job by a brother-in-law, computer generated land surveys, but it took every ounce of concentration I could force out of myself. My fellow co-workers knew I was a bit different and slow, but it was such a great company that they all reached out to me and still to this day, are very close friends. I messed up a lot on jobs, but then I found something that I was good at and became an expert in doing that kind of work and so I stood doing just that for over 16 years.

After a bitter divorce, I tried to broaden my knowledge and make more money with another company and moved to south Florida. A wrong move, for after 4 years I was let go, being that there wasn't any work for what I was doing for so long. I detested changes and was content on doing my job until I retired. I was petrified as to what to do next. The economy crashed and my field virtually disappeared, being that my job had to do with new construction and home purchases. I have been unemployed now for over two years. My fear of feeling alienated and starting a new career, meeting new people disables me.

Yet as I try to face this new challenge, I have discovered what may be the answer that I have been searching for. I found what is wrong with me. In my time off from work I started searching for what could be my hindrance in doing things that seem so simple to the majority. Add, ADHD, but nothing hit the target until I researched Autism and lo and behold, one aspect of Autism stood out as if the North Star itself was just a few feet from me, "Asperger's Syndrome." Not just one symptom, but all seem to hit right on, stories of others with this condition was as if they were reading my life story.

As tears trickled down my face, I felt as if a huge burden was lifted from me, I wasn't alone, there were and are others like me. The most important part is that now I have resources, personal experiences and information on how I can control this syndrome. Resources on how I can learn to live a normal life and another very important thing is that now I can give my family pamphlets, books to read so that they can start to understand me when they ask "what is wrong with you?" and have stood quiet in embarrassment because I never had an answer.

Finding answers when researching all about Aspergers, is like finding not only answers, but finally finding peace in my life as I know what my limitations are and learning to work around them. With new research being done on Autism and with new breakthroughs, I have hope that there won't be any more children on a corner of a school yard feeling left out, but sharing in all the fun as any other normal child. And that Aspergers comes to be understood and accepted as something in the workplace as normal as a wheelchair or crutches, thereby opening many doors for us and lastly keep them open regardless of our difference.

Best wishes to all,

Ray

***

Part One: Why get a diagnosis as an adult?

Before we talk about how to get a diagnosis as an adult, let us first explore the reasons you might want to. After all, you're not in school anymore. You don't need it for special education services. You don't need it to satisfy your parents. At this point, you've probably developed quite a few coping mechanisms to deal with many of the myriad problems of life as a person on the autistic spectrum. You know how to do small talk (a little), you know how to deal with people just enough to get by. You know what makes you happy (hopefully) and you stick to it. Your life might not be perfect but it works. So why get a diagnosis if you're in your 20s, 30s, 40s or beyond? Why bother to spend the time and energy?

First of all—curiosity. You've lived a long time knowing you act and think differently. You know the world seems to live according to different rules than you do. You are probably wondering, do I really have this Asperger's thing? Am I just trying to find an excuse for my laziness, or is this real? You might want to get a diagnosis just for validation. Validation can be a powerful emotional motivator. You know you've struggled all your life. You know you've had to work three times as hard as others to achieve what is sometimes only half as much. You know you're not lazy, crazy or stupid—or maybe you don't. But it sure would be nice to have a professional confirm it. Some adults feel having a diagnosis would be useful because it would be a way to "prove" themselves to their family and friends.

Rachel Cohen-Rottenberg is an adult woman with Asperger's who writes a wonderful, thought provoking blog about life with Asperger's at www.aspergerjourneys.com . In a May 2009 entry, Rachel discusses why she decided to seek a diagnosis of Asperger's as an adult:

"I don't think that many people understand the disorientation of not having a label, of not being able to give one's way of seeing a name. I wanted a label, and I wanted it from someone other than myself. I suppose it's my yearning to be part of the social world, to participate in that experience in which people mirror one another and help one another find identity. I'd always been the lone ranger, creating my own definitions, and asserting my own understanding. Except for my husband, I had never had a clear mirror, and when it came to an Asperger's diagnosis, I knew how deeply I needed one. I wanted someone else to call me an Aspie, to acknowledge my group identity, and to give me my name."

Rachel talks about the emotional longing to have a name for her troubles, her difficulties, her way of seeing the world. She speaks of wanting to belong somewhere. That is a common theme in many adults with Asperger's.

Accommodations at Work

Some adults need accommodations for their jobs. They have tried and tried to make it in the workplace as they are, but they have fallen short. Perhaps their workspace is too noisy. Perhaps they can't understand verbal directions and need things written down. Perhaps the overnight shift is too difficult and they need a transfer to daytime. Maybe they need a desk away from others so that the chaos of a busy workplace doesn't get to them, or want permission to wear headphones so they can focus. Maybe workplace politics are getting the best of them. With a diagnosis, some employers might be more open to alternate ways of communication that might work better and prevent some of the many misunderstandings that can come up with Asperger's.

Another woman with Asperger's in San Francisco writes about the issue on her blog, Aspie Talk, "It can be intimidating for people to reveal that they have Asperger's because employers and co-workers generally don't understand what it is, or hear that it is on the Autistic

214

spectrum and form unfavorable opinions. People with Asperger's in the workplace are often ostracized because they are unable to meet the overt or unspoken social expectations there. People with Asperger's often have overwhelming sensory experiences, and need accommodation, for example, to have dimmer lights, wear headphones so background noise is diminished and have a workplace setup that is more private."

With a proper diagnosis, you are entitled to accommodations in your workplace by law. The Americans With Disabilities Act mandates this. Your employer has to make "reasonable accommodations" for your disability. If you are having trouble keeping your job and performing your duties without accommodation, seeking a diagnosis of Asperger's might be helpful in this area.

Educational Accommodations

If you are in school, perhaps in college or you have gone back to school in mid-life, and you need accommodations for Asperger's symptoms, a diagnosis is helpful. Some accommodations that can be useful for an adult in college or grad school include things like:

- Extra time on tests

- Quiet rooms to take tests in that they are separate from where the class takes tests

- Tutors to help with difficult subjects

- Someone to take notes for you

- Even a peer mentor who can help with social issues on campus

There may be other unique issues you have to do that the disability office of a school can help you with. You will usually but not always need an official diagnosis to receive these services, however.

James Williams on the Positively Autism blog on the PsychologyToday.com website expands on the college and accommodation issue:

"Colleges offer a varying level of support and much of it depends on the size and funding of the Services for Students with Disabilities Office. On a small campus, the office could be minimally funded and offer very few basic services. However, it varies not only on size, but also on the commitment of the university to promote and accept the attendance of students with disabilities. Keep in mind, that the law says accommodations must be available to students with disabilities, but it does not specify the quality or size of those services. At my university, they offer several accommodations such as note-taking assistance, preferential seating, extended time, or alternate test site. In addition, they offer a weekly Asperger's syndrome/HFA group that is offered as part of the services available at the counseling center. Again, it varies school to school, but remember that just because an accommodation you want is not on their list, doesn't mean you can't ask for it and state your case."

Getting Other Services

Finally, one last reason that some might seek a diagnosis as an adult is to get services provided by the state or federal government for those with disabilities. Those may include things like a caseworker, who can help you get and coordinate other services; in home care, where someone will come in and help with things like cooking, cleaning, budgeting, exercise, and whatever other kind of help you might need in your daily life. You may also be eligible for disability payments if your Asperger's is determined so severe that you are not able to hold a job of any kind.

Lisa Jo Rudy of the About.com Autism site further expands on why getting a diagnosis as an adult is important:

"Diagnosis can provide a framework for labeling, understanding and learning about behavioral and emotional challenges that have perhaps seemed inexplicable up to this point. This can diminish shame, lead to a greater sense of community and begin the process of learning to live more adaptively with an Asperger's brain. It may also help others in your life understand and respond differently."

She also gives ten reason why adults who think they may have Asperger's should seek out a diagnosis.

1. Career Reasons

If you never seem to get the job that reflects your abilities despite your education level. You keep getting passed over for promotions or you seem under employed and office politics bewilders you. It just could be AS.

2. Friendships Reasons

You have always had a tough time making friends. And if you make a few, they don't seem to stay around too long. Or you share less of a personal bond than a bond that relates to a particular activity that you share. Maybe this is related to AS also.

3. The Reason you "Obsess" on Certain Topics

Maybe you have been thought of as fanatical or obsessive throughout your life but you think of yourself as just interested in one special subject. Maybe you have been told that you go on obsessively about a topic to the point that you bore others. Are you right or are others right? Should you be expanding your interests? It may help you to know if you have AS.

4. Socially You're Not Making It

Parties, get-togethers, social events where you meet people—do they make you feel like a fish out of water? But these are the essential places to make friends, meet your future spouse, or schmooze for that important business contact. But if they are always too loud for you to enjoy, you never know what to wear, you cannot carry on a conversation and you cannot figure out how to take part and have fun—the problem may be AS.

5. Romance Reasons

Dating baffles you. It never works out. Yes you try but you never seem to get to first base. Let's face it. It's tough for many people. But is it tougher for you just because you have had bad luck or is Asperger's a part of the equation?

6. Lights, Cameras, Action! Oh No!

You really would like to go to a concert or the mall— even the grocery store! But all those lights, the people, the hustle and bustle. How do others stand it? You would like to be comfortable at sporting events and take part in ordinary activities like other people do. The problem could be AS and part of the solution could be starting with getting a diagnosis.

7. To Make it Easier to Get Through School

Wish a formal diagnosis of Asperger's syndrome, a whole world of educational accommodations will likely open up to you. You may be able to get more time to take tests, special tutors may be offered, perhaps you can take tests or exams in a quieter room or get special training to help with interviews. These doors will not open for you without a formal diagnosis.

8. To Solve a Problem in an Important Relationship

Maybe a special person in your life has suggested that you get a diagnosis. Perhaps they see something that you don't. Maybe some aspect of your behavior is driving them crazy. Maybe they are right, maybe not. But a professional can sort it all out for you.

9. A Diagnosis of Asperger's Syndrome May Be the Key to Getting Services You Need

With a diagnosis of Asperger's syndrome, you may qualify for a whole host of service you may never have realized exist. From help with job counseling to housing assistance to a variety of local, state and federal services, accommodations and supports.

10. A Diagnosis of Asperger's Syndrome Can Open New Doors to Friendships and Community

Have you felt different your whole life? There are a lot of support groups with people just like you. An entire community of adults with Asperger's who act, think and understand how you tick. A formal diagnosis may be just what you need to motivate you to join a group, make some friends, get some support and connect with the community.

Once you've identified the problem, you can start looking for a solution or proper accommodations to help each of these issues.

Resistance to or Problems with Getting a Diagnosis

There are many good reasons adults with AS may want to seek a formal diagnosis, but it is not for everyone. Some adults with possible AS are very resistant to the idea.

1. Some adults do not feel that there is anything wrong with them.

They can't believe, or they don't want to believe, that they are different from their peers. They want to blend in, they want to be "normal," and they don't want to hear anything that threatens their belief of their normality. Some are depressed over their differences and turn to video games, online role playing games, or other special interests to drown out their worries and fears.

Many parents worry about their adult children who don't seem to be able to accept that they have special challenges and might need some extra guidance to succeed. They want their kids to see a counselor, get a job, make friends. It can be very difficult to help someone who does not want to be helped. Sometimes the adult with Asperger's is not ready or able to face up to the fact that his or her difference has a name and is a life-long, permanent thing.

Of course, there are positives to having AS as well. but they can be hard to see when all you know is how socially miserable you are and all you can think about is the areas you don't function so well in. Some adults are in denial simply because they don't want to think of themselves as different. As long as they are managing to lead lives that are meaningful and enjoyable to them, as long as they are able to be productive in some way, this is fine; there is no reason to get a diagnosis if you

220

are not having problems functioning. If you are having issues, though, getting help is advisable.

2. Money

Depending on whom you see, what kind of doctor, and what kind of insurance you have, getting a diagnosis can be a very expensive proposition. Many adults put off or avoid getting a formal diagnosis for reasons of cost.

3. Satisfied the way they are

Many adults might have self-diagnosed themselves using information found on the Internet or in books and are happy with this self-knowledge. They know they have AS, they know why they're different, and this is enough. They don't feel it is worth the trouble to have a professional back them up on it. They know it's true and that is all that matters to them.

4. No qualified doctors locally

In many areas, there may be very few doctors or psychologists with knowledge of Asperger's. In that case, it can be hard to find someone knowledgeable enough to make a diagnosis of Asperger's in an adult. Asperger's is much more commonly diagnosed in kids than adults, and it might be hard to find a doctor who knows enough about the presentation of Asperger's in adults to make a proper diagnosis.

Carien's Story

Craig,

You asked me if I could tell "our" story for your book. The problem is that I don't know for sure if our 30 year old son Jeff has Aspersers. It is possible that he has ADHD (the Inattentive Type). We won't know what his disorder is until he is tested and diagnosed.

I mentioned in my email to you that Jeff only contacts us when he is completely down and out. Jeff moved back home a week before Christmas because he had no place to stay, no job and no money. Our agreement was that, if he wanted to stay for a long period of time, to get back on his feet, we would help him as much as we could, but he would have to find a job, at least try his best to find a job. He had agreed.

Per computer he found a temporary job as a technical tech assistant, locally. He said the job was ok, but boring. Unfortunately this job only lasted two weeks.

Even though he avoided talking to his dad during this time, he and I were able to have some communication during that time, but after the temp. job was finished, he completely "shut down".

He started to avoid us, barely any communication whatsoever for about 10 days or more. He locked himself up in his room most of the time, only coming out when my husband and I weren't there or were asleep.

He knew he had to go and find another job, but didn't try. We left him alone and didn't mention it. However, one morning, when he thought no one was home, he found me sitting at the kitchen table. I greeted him, fixed breakfast and asked him what his plans were. He said he didn't want to talk, and didn't want to deal with getting a job, and getting his life in order yet. I didn't get a chance to respond, for he locked himself up again.

He suddenly left early the next morning, without saying goodbye or where is was going, leaving a few clothes and his computer behind. He left in his old car with a little money of the 14 day temp. job. I have a feeling that he is living in his car somewhere, either in Mississippi, Louisiana or any of the other southern states.

After I left him many voice messages telling him that I am very concerned about him, he finally text messaged me yesterday to say that he is fine, (and that was all he wrote).

I found out that we have a Mental Health Clinic here locally, where he can be evaluated inexpensively, one pays according to income, but as long as Jeff stays "on the run", and doesn't want to be helped, there is not much we can do.

Needlessly to say, stress in your book that parents pay attention to the behavior of their children, and have their children tested when something just doesn't seem right. When they are over 18 years of age, it is too late when the child doesn't want to be tested or helped.

There were so many "reasons" in our household explaining Jeff's behavior, that we never saw the forest through the trees. Looking back, and knowing now what we didn't know then, it is obvious something else was going on with him beside the "reasons".

Thank you for all your newsletters, which I'll continue to read, thank you for all the good work you do, and best of luck with your new book.

Best regards,

Carien

***

Part Two: How to Get a Diagnosis of Asperger's as an Adult

The symptoms of Asperger's in an adult can present quite differently than the symptoms of Asperger's in a child. Most family doctors are trained—sometimes—to recognize autistic spectrum symptoms in a child, but few know what it looks like in an adult. Since most AS diagnoses come when a child is younger, most often when they start school and the social challenges become more obvious, obtaining an Asperger's diagnosis for an adult can sometimes be quite challenging.

One reason it is harder to diagnose an adult with Asperger's is that by the time most adults reach a more advanced age, they have picked up lots of coping skills along the way. They have learned to hide or mask some of their more different AS like traits to try to get along with the neurotypical outside world. This does not mean they don't still have problems coping and functioning with the world, however. It just means they have learned to hide it better and can "turn off" some issues some of the time—but not all of the time. A skilled psychologist or practitioner will be able to see behind the mask the learned coping skills create to the problems that still lie beneath; and will realize a diagnosis is still more than appropriate, based on past history and present remaining problems. If the doctor you are seeing does not seem too knowledgeable about Asperger's in adults and tells you that you couldn't have it because you are "functioning too well," it is okay and recommended, even, to try to seek out a different clinician with a little bit more knowledge and experience.

Not all practitioners go by exactly the same criteria, or have the same level of knowledge. Some only know the traditional definitions of autism, and think that if you are verbal and communicate well, if you have any friends at all, that you can't possibly have an autism spectrum disorder such as Asperger's. Such people fail to differentiate between symptoms of more classical autism and those of Asperger's. Again, if you get someone like this, feel free to seek a second opinion from someone with more experience.

What are the criteria for a diagnosis of Asperger's?

In order to receive a diagnosis of Asperger's syndrome, you must meet the following criteria, as set out by the Diagnostic and Statistical Manual of Mental Disorders, or DSM, which is the official handbook of what is a disorder and what is not.

From the Autreat.com site, printed in the DSM IV:

(I) "Qualitative impairment in social interaction, as manifested by at least two of the following:

(A) marked impairments in the use of multiple nonverbal behaviors such as eye-to-eye gaze, facial expression, body posture, and gestures to regulate social interaction

(B) failure to develop peer relationships appropriate to developmental level

(C) a lack of spontaneous seeking to share enjoyment, interest or achievements with other people, (e.g. by a lack of showing, bringing, or pointing out objects of interest to other people)

(D) lack of social or emotional reciprocity

(II) Restricted repetitive & stereotyped patterns of behavior, interests and activities, as manifested by at least one of the following:

   (A) encompassing preoccupation with one or more stereotyped and restricted patterns of interest that is abnormal either in intensity or focus

   (B) apparently inflexible adherence to specific, nonfunctional routines or rituals

   (C) stereotyped and repetitive motor mannerisms (e.g. hand or finger flapping or twisting, or complex whole-body movements)

   (D) persistent preoccupation with parts of objects

(III) The disturbance causes clinically significant impairments in social, occupational, or other important areas of functioning.

(IV) There is no clinically significant general delay in language (e.g. single words used by age 2 years, communicative phrases used by age 3 years)

(V) There is no clinically significant delay in cognitive development or in the development of age-appropriate self help skills, adaptive behavior (other than in social interaction) and curiosity about the environment in childhood.

(VI) Criteria are not met for another specific Pervasive Developmental Disorder or Schizophrenia."

If you fit the above symptoms, then you probably have Asperger's syndrome. A well qualified professional will be able to tell you more definitively.

What kind of medical professionals diagnose Asperger's?

Your primary care doctor may be able to recommend someone versed in Asperger's, or may not be able to. Many psychologists and psychiatrists are able to make this diagnosis. Your local autism society can probably refer you to someone who has enough experience with AS to make an Asperger's diagnosis.

How is a diagnosis made?

There are many different ways that a diagnosis can be made. Some clinicians will interview you and look for tell-tale symptoms like having difficulty making friends, using social language, using overly pedantic or formal language, having high intelligence (not all people with AS do but many will), demonstration of special interests, empathy, insight into others' feelings, and other similar classic Asperger's traits.

Some will administer tests and scales to judge the number of Asperger's traits you have. Many will want to interview your parents for their take on what your childhood and development was like. Some will want to give you neuro-cognitive testing. There are many different tests that measure Asperger's symptoms, but there is no one right or wrong, gold standard test. The diagnosis of Asperger's remains a somewhat subjective field.

Dr. Shana Nichols of the Lindner Center for Autism on Long Island, New York diagnoses many teens and adults with autism and Asperger's. She often gives an IQ test, since normal to high IQ scores are something that come up a lot with AS. She tests the adaptive skills of patients, testing their ability to manage complex social situations. She also interviews parents if available for their take on the person's history.

Lisa Jo Rudy of About.com interviewed Nichols to learn more about the diagnosis process.

"Nichols administers the ADOS Module IV. ADOS is the autism diagnostic observation schedule, and module four is for high-functioning verbal young adults and adults. Along with the ADI, it allows doctors to look carefully at social and communication skills and behavior. For example, says Nichols, the tests look at such questions as "Can you have a reciprocal social conversation? Are you interested in the examiner's thoughts and feelings? Do you demonstrate insight into relationships? Do you use appropriate non-verbal gestures and facial expressions? Do you have odd or over-focused interests?" The tests allow doctors to attach a grade in each domain to determine whether the patient meets the criteria for AS."

Sometimes people can be diagnosed and assessed in a single session and sometimes it takes many, depending on whom you see. Sometimes the cost is covered by your insurance, and sometimes it isn't, depending, again, on whom you see.

Ruling out other conditions

A doctor will want to make sure you do not have other similar conditions, whose symptoms can overlap with Asperger's. Some of these conditions may include the following:

> **Social anxiety**: severe anxiety around other people.

> **Auditory processing disorder**: trouble processing language; people talk and you hear them but don't understand the words.

> **Nonverbal learning disorder**: trouble using and understanding nonverbal language; similar to AS but with different features.

➢ **Attention deficit disorder**: trouble maintaining attention and focus, often hyperactivity.

➢ **Obsessive compulsive disorder**: thoughts that repeat in your head over and over again; a high degree of anxiety and worry; feeling the need to perform certain actions over and over again in order to feel safe. Many people with AS have features of this disorder, but OCD and AS are two separate diagnoses.

➢ **Selective mutism**: when you can only talk in certain situations, such as when you feel comfortable with the person, or with your family; inability to talk in many social situations.

These are just some of the illnesses whose symptoms in some ways can mimic Asperger's. Your doctor will want to test you to make sure to differentiate both from these and other kinds of pervasive developmental disorders. Asperger's is on the autistic spectrum, which means there are different kinds of and degrees of autism. Sometimes if an adult has some of the symptoms of Asperger's and some of classic autism, and can't really be put in one category, the diagnosis will be pervasive development disorder, not otherwise specified; it's basically a way of saying that you're on the autism spectrum, but they don't know exactly where to place you. It is a very similar thing to having AS. Different doctors will use these labels in different ways. Some will be more likely to diagnose AS. Others may slap a PDD-NOS label on you, and so on. But they mean very similar things.

High Functioning Autism and Asperger's: What is the difference?

HFA and Asperger's are very similar in presentation, especially by the time you get to adulthood. Generally speaking, the only difference is that people with HFA had a language delay as a child, and people with AS didn't. Otherwise, they overlap quite a bit.

What kinds of questions are asked in an interview to diagnose Asperger's?

There is unfortunately no one standardized scale used to diagnose everyone with Asperger's. Several different kinds are used. Most tests or scales will ask things like the following (most of which can be found on the Australian Scale for Asperger's syndrome):

Social and emotional abilities:

✓ Do you understand other people's motivations and intents?

✓ Or are you kind of oblivious?

Communication abilities:

✓ Do you interpret language literally?

✓ Do you have good eye contact?

✓ Do you have an unusual tone of voice, perhaps somewhat flat?

Cognitive skills:

✓ Do you read books for information but dislike fiction books?

✓ Do you have a great memory for facts and details that happened long ago?

These are some things that are commonly seen in people and adults with Asperger's.

Specific interests:

✓ Do you collect mounds of information and statistics on a particular topic?

Movement Skills:

✓ Do you have poor motor coordination?

Other:

✓ Do you have high anxiety?

✓ Unusual sensory sensitivities?

✓ Unusual body movements or facial tics?

Most clinicians will interview you about your life, and in the course of the interview and assessment, attempt to answer the above questions. You may be asked to manipulate objects to assess your motor skills, or to put together puzzles or other such tasks to further determine the way your brain works and solves problems. There are many different ways to go about assessing Asperger's; in the end, they all serve the same purpose, though.

Part Three: After the Diagnosis: Coming to Terms with Asperger's Syndrome

So, you jumped through all the hoops. You decided to seek out a diagnosis. You found a psychologist or professional who could diagnose you. And you went through all the testing. This can be a stressful process. In the end, you have joined the club and were given a diagnosis of Asperger's. Now the hard part starts—dealing with your emotions and feelings about the diagnosis.

Most people will have a large variety of reactions to this, which are perfectly normal and common. Some people feel very relieved. Finally, they know what is "wrong" with them, and why they are different. They can start trying to accept who they are and build a new life based on this new self-knowledge. It can be a very empowering and releasing thing to realize that you are okay the way you are. You're not broken or diseased or crazy; you just have a different way of looking at the world. Your brain is just wired a little differently than everyone else's.

Others feel very worried and agitated. They don't want to have a label. They don't want to be seen as "sick." They feel that the diagnosis is something of a life sentence. They feel they will never have a normal life now. The news can make them very depressed. Difficulties they might have thought they could grow out of, they now realize might be with them for a long time. Perhaps the process has illustrated to them just how different and isolated from other people they are. Their task is to find a way to come to terms with their diagnosis and see what they still can give to the world, instead of focusing on what they are lacking.

Some are in denial and refuse to believe that the diagnosis is true. Some want to tell their friends, family and co-workers immediately. Others make a pact not to tell anyone, ever. Some will share the news with close friends but guard it very privately in other situations, like work.

There may be a sense of wonder at having everything fall into place, or a sense of shame at being different. Or it might not mean much to you either way, as you figure you are the same person you were before the diagnosis.

Sometimes, there is a sense of profound loss. The person realizes just how much of normal social life they have missed out on due to their difficulties. They realize how big the gap is between them and everyone else. Their increased awareness of social matters spurs them to want to increase their efforts to make friends, but they run into brick walls and fail. They become acutely aware of the fact that no matter how hard they try, they always seem to be alone. This can cause a sense of despair. The process of trying to accept yourself as someone with this unique set of challenges can be a long one. You have to have a whole new way of thinking of yourself and the way you function in the world.

A.J. Mahari of the Canadian based Asperger Adults Support Network echoes this theme in many of the essays on her website. She is an adult with Asperger's who was diagnosed late in life.

A.J. says, "It is difficult, taxing, and tiring trying to pretend to be "normal". It is also heart-wrenching in terms of awakening to the reality of difference. I still do not understand how others feel when they socialize, for example, and try as I might to understand this, I just don't. Knowing this is lonely. Knowing this is isolating.

What can be changed? Can I learn to feel in relation to others as opposed to just feeling stuff inside of myself that I've come to know is cut-off from others and has little or nothing to do with them? Can I learn to understand, feel and derive some pleasure out of socialization? I rather doubt it. I know though that I can continue to learn how to "pretend" more effectively to be "normal". This allows me to "connect" with others or work with others and interact with others but in so doing, I awake even more to my loneliness because with this increased exposure to others comes a much more profound and deeper understanding of my differences. Insert hit brick wall here."

A.J. talks very profoundly about the struggle to connect with others and her increasing awareness of how big the gap between her and other people is. After her diagnosis, she does a lot of soul searching and tries to figure out who, exactly, she is, and what she is supposed to do with what she has. That can often be a difficult question. Where do we fit in the world?

"Awakening to despair. Awakening to an aching-longing sense of loss. A loss that represents my isolation. An isolation that has existed all my life and only been known or realized in stages, or to differing degrees as I grew older. Suddenly it is screamingly—loud. It is obvious and abundantly clear—now what? I am a 44 year old egocentric child, socially lost and too busy inside myself to appreciate the views and feelings of others. What am I supposed to do with this?"

After the diagnosis, one is left to figure out new ways of giving and ordering meaning to their world. A little self-knowledge can go a long way.

One Woman's Story: Getting a Diagnosis at 21

It is useful to learn about experiences directly from those who experience them. To that end, here is an account by a young woman who did not receive a diagnosis of Asperger's until she was almost all the way through college, at age 21. She explains the process, and the thoughts and feelings involved.

Anonymous

I always knew there was something different about me, but I didn't know what. I would always tell guidance counselors, parents, etc. that I felt like I was on a different planet from everyone else. Nothing about the way I thought, felt and acted seemed to be like my peers. They just told me I was quirky and would grow out of it. Not to worry about it. But I knew it was something more than that.

I finally got my answer in my junior year of college. I was watching a movie on TV about a young boy with autism who used facilitated communication to talk with others. I looked up the topic on the Internet and started reading about autism. I checked out a dozen or more books from the library about autism and Asperger's. By the time a year had passed I'd consumed everything I could get my hands on about autism, numbering almost forty books; I especially liked reading memoirs by people with Asperger's or autism, because I could relate to them so much.

Despite this all, I still didn't have an official diagnosis. I had to wait about 18 months for that. I went back and forth in my head many times, trying to decide if I really had it or not. I felt like while I fit the textbook definition of many of the traits, there were a few glaring things I felt did not fit. I felt I was too emotional to have AS, for one thing; I felt and expressed my emotions very strongly. A lot of the literature about AS says that people with AS have little or no affect, and that wasn't me. Also, the literature talks about little empathy, and I knew that wasn't me, either. These turned out to be misconceptions; people with AS have emotions and empathy like everyone else, they just show it differently.

When I finally did go see a psychologist to inquire about the possibility of Asperger's, I was nervous. I didn't know what he would say, if I would be taken seriously or not. To my utter surprise, after talking to me for an hour at the end of the first session, he said to me, "You're a textbook case of Asperger's." I was stunned. A year and a half of worry and anguish over whether or not I had it, and he was able to say this so decisively after only knowing me for an hour? Mostly, though, I was relieved. My difficulties finally made sense. I could finally fit myself into a framework that made sense. There was a reason why I thought differently. Now I could try to find others who thought the same way, and learn ways to try to overcome some of my difficulties! It felt like being able to truly breathe for the first time; talking to the psychologist, he really seemed to "get" everything I was experiencing. He was able to describe the way my mind functioned better than anyone else ever had. It was a relief to be understood in this way.

My parents became a lot more understanding after I received the diagnosis. They were able to see where I was coming from more. I met other people my age with AS and started to feel a sense of self-acceptance for the first time in my life. A sense of belonging somewhere. So for me, getting a diagnosis of Asperger's as an adult, at age 21, was a very liberating and positive thing. Some people will ask why it matters once you're an adult, but I would say the self-knowledge it gives you sets you free.

***

These themes of accidental self-discovery of Asperger's, internal debate and wondering if it applies to you, and a sense of relief after diagnosis are very common in many adults with Asperger's.

Finally, we will look at one final perspective, from Barbara Kirby, who is the founder of the very comprehensive Asperger's website OASIS:
(http://aspergersyndrome.org):

"To come to a diagnosis of Asperger's syndrome in adulthood, as I did, at the age of 40, can initially be both a relief and a nightmare. The relief, as I experienced it, had all to do with finally understanding so much about all that was so difficult and painful in my life.

The nightmare was the process it took to integrate how much I had suffered without an understanding of why I had been so alone (always felt different) most of my life and why trying to relate to others or be social was extremely difficult most of the time, if not impossible, for me at other times.

Without any understanding of what was really behind most of my relational difficulties I was left to feel, time and time again, like I was "less than", like a failure. I experienced this as being "unlikable and unlovable" Feeling this way lead me to feel very alienated. I had spent most of my life frantically searching for what was "wrong" with me. My family, peers, and society at large gave me endless messages that I was not okay.

Not understanding this very pervasive aspect of myself left me unable to really understand who I was. Without this knowledge of my "self" I was lost and in a great deal of pain for much of my first 40 years of life. Not knowing why I was the way I was, the way that I am, still, caused me to try to be whatever others told me I "should" be. This was torture. This is the epitome of being lost. I was alienated from my very self by the expectations and judgments of others.

My lack of being "what others expected me to be" along with my lack of knowing what others have always expected that I "should" know based upon my age or intelligence was literally crazy-making."

One of the most important tasks that adults with AS have, especially the newly diagnosed, is to re-learn the messages that society has taught them about their self-worth and about what kinds of ways of being in the world are okay. They have to come to realize that everyone has their own way of doing things; that they are not deficient, wrong, stupid, lazy or crazy just because they do things a different way. Self-acceptance is a huge task.

A Note on Self Diagnosis

A lot of people do not feel the need to get formally diagnosed. They have done the research on the Internet about Asperger's, perhaps talked to others with AS, and are fairly certain that they have it. Sometimes just knowing it exists is enough to set their minds at ease. They don't feel the need to pay for or take the time to get a formal diagnosis from a doctor. This is okay, too. There are many tools you can use on the Internet that will ask you questions about your past and present, your way of thinking, acting, coping etc. to help you decide if you think you might have Asperger's. Some are better than others but most are pretty comprehensive. These should not, of course, be substituted for a medical diagnosis if you need such a thing for work, school or other situations. But they can be helpful for your own knowledge and education.

In this chapter, we have talked about why a person would want to get a diagnosis of Asperger's. What the potential problems could be to doing this. How to go about doing it. What the diagnostic process is like and what feelings to expect after receiving an Asperger's diagnosis. It is by no means an easy process to even contemplate a diagnosis of Asperger's syndrome, as an adult or any other time. There are a lot of difficult feelings that go along with it. The process can be time consuming and expensive. It can be hard to find someone knowledgeable to diagnose you. But in the end, it seems a worthwhile thing to do. Self-knowledge is everything; and once you know what you're dealing with, you can start to figure out ways to make it better.

Angelina's Story

My name is Angelina. I'm a 48 year old African American woman who has not been diagnosed with Asperger's syndrome, but I do have many of the traits of this disorder. Early in life I knew I was different. As a small child I would rock, speak in my own language, and I hated being held or touched by anyone including family members. I had and still have strange tick-like behavior.

Many people thought I was retarded but, with my level of intelligence, retardation does not fit. I graduated salutatorian from business school, was awarded aide of the year in 2009 twice, and I have a license to sell life insurance.

Because of my poor social skills, the only people who will hire me are low income jobs. I still could not figure out what was wrong with me. Then I heard of Asperger's syndrome and decided to do some research on the internet. When I listen to those who have been diagnosed I think to myself, they sound just like me. The sad thing about having autism is, you look normal so your disorder is invisible to other people's eyes. So therefore, me and people like me have been subjected to unbelievable cruelty.

Because of the way I've been treated my entire life, I have great anger and resentment for people. I'm very religious so the bible has helped me to be more forgiving. But I am still constantly confused by what other people are saying, thinking or feeling, and as a result I have been bullied relentlessly as a child and had altercations at work. I find that I'm much happier when contact with people is kept to a minimum.

I feel like I'm trapped in a world I don't understand. NOBODY understands how I feel except my heavenly father and people who have Asperger's. The only thing holding me back now for getting a diagnosis is I have no medical coverage so I don't have the financial resources to get diagnosed. But when I do it will be a great relief to me to finally know what's wrong and to get the help which is long overdue. I say this with tears and hope.

Sincerely,

Angelina

***

Cherie's Story

I am 56 yrs old, been married happily for 25 years with two beautiful daughters. Our second daughter who will be turning 21 in a few months was our "challenging" child. At first we thought it was the 2nd child syndrome or sibling rivalry. By 18 months old she was headstrong, with her own agenda.

I read parenting books and took classes in active parenting with no success in teaching her the rights and wrongs, that there were consequences for wrong/inappropriate behavior, etc. She did whatever she wanted to do despite the consequences. Trying to make her do something such as apologizing, doing a chore, etc. was the biggest mistake. These incidents always got ugly and tense causing a lot of tension in the family and a lose-lose situation. She would retreat to her room, stomping and yelling, slamming the door and then sit in her room and weep.

I could never understand why she wept when she was so obviously the one who was breaking the rules, etc. She never seemed to "get it", whatever we were trying to teach her. Her grandmother went to her grave not understanding why her granddaughter never acted happy with any gifts she received from her, rather emotionless, and then wouldn't thank her. The only emotion she was really good at displaying growing up was anger, or frowning. We used to refer to her privately as our "rain cloud". We tried "tough love" discipline in her early teens. This only escalated the problem, making her totally uncooperative.

Out of desperation we finally took her to counseling. She had to be physically escorted into the building each session. She spent the next 6 months letting us know in every way she could that she "hated" us for this. She spent many sessions not speaking to the psychologist and holding back. Those were some really dark days for our family. The counselor called me and asked us to come in and speak to her without our daughter. She then went on to tell us that she had opened a small line of communication with our daughter and that she thought she had Asperger's Syndrome. She wanted to test her for this but had to order the test. During the next few months, the counseling continued but the test didn't come in. In the meantime, the counselor who was pregnant became high risk and was ordered to bed rest, causing our therapy to abruptly end. There was no question about starting over with a new counselor, that was just too painful to consider doing to the entire family. We opted to wait for her to come back. But in the end, by the time she came back 6 months later the fight had gone out of my husband to make her go back to therapy.

241

Our daughter had just started treating us nicely again and her behavior was actually improved somewhat, so the therapy went by the wayside. That was 6 years ago and I have watched my daughter slowly mature. There are still areas that she still doesn't "get it" and I think that will always be that way. I have never told her that she might have Asperger's Syndrome and now regret it as I feel I lost my window to tell her. My husband is adamant that she not know since she was never formally diagnosed and that might make her feel like she's "broken". She definitely thought that when we put her in counseling, that we thought she was broken. Anyway, she still doesn't communicate much with us.

To this day, I couldn't tell you how she feels about anything. She has never, ever expressed her emotions on any subject. I also know she doesn't confide with her friends either. This makes me sad as I feel there's such a void between us. I typically get yes or no answers and if I push for explanations she really shuts down and either starts yelling at me "I don't know" or just gets up and leaves. I have been reading your newsletters for the past 2 years and it has helped me tremendously. I am beginning to understand my daughter better. I still don't know how to bridge the chasm between us and I still don't know how to get her to understand something she doesn't comprehend. But I do know that she does have feelings, emotions inside that she just isn't showing us. I still get very frustrated with her for being so "controlling", but at least I understand why. For the longest time I didn't understand how she rationalizes, but now I'm starting to understand that her comprehension is totally different from us. I now know that she has a lot of anxiety that we don't know about which displays itself through seemingly stubbornness, controlling, or rude behavior. This has helped to alleviate a lot of my anger towards her behavior.

I used to feel guilty for my love/hate feelings towards my own daughter. Now I no longer feel the hate. I understand she has a disorder. I only regret that we hadn't followed through with her counseling. I would love some direction on what to do with her tentative diagnosis and how or if we should tell her. I would love for her to seek her own help, but she was never cooperative, so that leads me to think she would never seek help on her own. Thank you so very much for your newsletter, you have given me a whole new perspective about my daughter. I now have a better idea what goes on in her mind. She also never shares daily experiences or her life with us. Is this normal?

Cherie

[Note from the author: I have been in contact with Cherie. I suggested she find a new therapist that specializes in Asperger's syndrome and slowly work with her daughter to encourage her to seek counseling]

***

10. Therapy Options

When you have problems in your life functioning in different areas, sometimes you don't even know if you need help or not. You think to yourself, I've always done things this way. It's not perfect, but it works well enough. I've gotten through all of my life without help, why should I get help now?

There are many reasons why an adult with Asperger's might resist or be unsure about therapy. They have had years and years to develop coping mechanisms that work for them. They may still experience difficulty but they feel that things work well enough and how could anyone possibly help them or improve upon what they have already done? They might feel a sense of bitterness or resentment, even, that they had to get so far on their own without the kind of help they wanted, and figure it's far too late to start now. Or maybe they do genuinely want help but don't know that it's out there or available. They don't know where to look, or how to afford it. They need help with transportation, or they don't like the first counselor they see. There are a lot of roadblocks to getting therapy. Most people don't associate therapy with adults as much as kids and don't know it's possible. This chapter talks about the possible therapies available for adults with Asperger's.

Why therapy?

A lot of adults with Asperger's function quite well despite their difficulties. They may ask more questions than others at work, might talk in a stilted manner and get upset more easily than others, but they can carry out all of the functions required of them without too much difficulty. But in their personal life, they are not happy; they want more connection with others, they feel lonely and unsatisfied. Many suffer from depression over the lack of ability to get close to others. Many have a lot of debilitating anxiety. Therapy can help with these things. Others are more affected. Their sensory issues are getting in the way of their lives. They can't be in noisy environments at all, can't stand the feel of clothes on their body, can't process information without getting overwhelmed. *Sensory integration therapy* can be useful for this. Others need help with basic life skills, cooking, cleaning, time management, money management. *Occupational therapy* can help with this. Some people just need counseling on how to deal with everyday situations in their lives. Others need *social skills classes* and instruction, because they never got it when they were younger or else just need more. There are lots of reasons adults with Asperger's can benefit from different types of therapy.

Common Reasons Adults Refuse Therapy

Why are some adults with Asperger's resistant or hesitant to the idea of getting therapy? This is a common question asked by many loved ones of adults with AS. There can be several reasons.

1. Denial of diagnosis

Some newly diagnosed adults with AS don't believe they have anything wrong with them and therefore nothing requires fixing. This kind of resistance can be

245

hard to overcome and it is best to wait until the adult feels a need to work on their issues themselves.

2. They don't know that help is available

A lot is made out of therapies for kids and teenagers with autism spectrum disorders but very few people ever talk about treatments for adults. A lot of adults might not know there is help for their sensory issues, social gaffes or anxiety.

3. They aren't comfortable with their first therapist

It takes many tries sometimes to find a therapist you are comfortable with. You also have to think of what kind of therapy—talk therapy, cognitive therapy, analysis, and so on—you want to be in. Some kinds will work better than others and suit your temperament. You might have to try a few different therapists and a couple of different orientations before something clicks for you.

4. They don't have enough money

It is important to find a therapist that is covered by your insurance. This may require looking around a little. If you have Medicare, it can sometimes be harder to find qualified professionals that are covered by Medicare. Occupational therapists are not always covered, but sometimes are. Co-pays might be too high for the person's budget.

5. They think they can cope on their own

As mentioned earlier, a lot of adults feel like this is all stuff they've dealt with all their lives, so why bother getting help now when they've done fine until now? They don't realize how much easier of a time they

246

might have with help or don't believe that help is possible. Some men have more masculine attitudes and think that they should just tough out their issues on their own. Some might think that therapy will be too much work.

6. Going into strange buildings makes some people uncomfortable

Some adults with AS might not want to spend all that time in an office building if they are afraid to leave home or have sensitivities to noises or smells that they do not want to encounter. If you can find someone who does phone appointments or even home visits—not that there many of them these days—that would work better. Or perhaps the therapist would be willing to meet in a neutral place such as outside.

7. Lack of transportation

Depending on their living situation, getting to a therapist can be too cumbersome, especially if they have to use public transportation. Public transit can be overwhelming, with lots of unpredictable noises, people, smells and chaos and the adult with AS who doesn't drive might not want to use it any more than they have to.

So, as you can see, there are many reasons that lots of adults with AS don't take advantage of all of the opportunities out there that could possibly help them. As the loved one of someone with AS, if you are aware of these reasons, you can try to find solutions to the problems and ways to work around them so that if therapy is something that could benefit them, they will be able to access it. Maybe you could help them research therapists who would be good for them, research the different types available in your area, help with transportation, and just

247

generally help educate them about what is out there. Ease any anxieties about what they will have to do or say and what will be expected of them.

Overview of different types of therapy

There are many different types of therapy available to adults with Asperger's. First, we need to split it into different categories.

- Psychotherapy: which can be mainly divided into talk therapy and cognitive therapy or behavior therapy

- Occupational Therapy: different kinds of including sensory integration therapy, is another.

Both of these can be very useful to adults with Asperger's.

Psychotherapy

Psychotherapy is the classic kind of therapy most people think of when they think of therapy. You sit with a therapist and talk to them about your problems. What they do with the problems can differ greatly depending on their orientation, though. Some will sit and help you process your issues. "What does that mean to you?" "What does that feel like? How do you feel when you talk about that?" Some will try to give you direction and orientation. "Do you think it would have worked better if you'd done X? What do you think Billy was thinking when you said that?"

Beyond that, you have the *cognitive model*, which says that most of your problems result from faulty thinking and that the thought processes need to be changed. You have the *behavioral model*, which follows Skinner's behaviorism theory and says that all problems are a result of aberrant behaviors; furthermore that people can be trained not to engage in these behaviors by providing rewards or other such incentives.

And you have the *psychoanalysis model* which bases its work on Freud's theories, and involves spending a lot of time talking about your childhood, dreams, and the symbolism of various things.

One thing that is important in all kinds of therapy is to have empathy. You have to feel that the therapist understands you and understands what you are going through. You have to have a feeling of connection for any kind of therapy to work.

Sometimes *group therapy* is used. Anywhere from 5 to 20 people meet as a group to talk about their (usually shared) issues, to listen to each other and give each other feedback. This can be helpful for some adults with Asperger's who are learning how to communicate better with others and want to practice their social skills with others; it is best done with others who have similar issues, though.

Allpsych.com describes group therapy this way, "Often group therapy is utilized, where individuals suffering from similar illnesses or having similar issues meet together with one or two therapists. Group sizes differ, ranging from three or four to upwards of 15 or 20, but the goals remain the same. The power of group is due to the need in all of us to belong, feel understood, and know that there is hope. All of these things make group as powerful as it is. Imagine feeling alone, scared, misunderstood, unsupported, and unsure of the future; then imagine entering a group of people with similar issues who have demonstrated success, who can understand the feelings you have, who support and encourage you, and who accept you as an important part of the group. It can be overwhelming in a very positive way and continues to be the second most utilized treatment after individual therapy."

249

What is required for a good match with a psychotherapist?

1. You feel comfortable with the therapist; you feel the therapist has empathy for you and can express it in a way you can understand.

2. The therapist is non-judgmental; she or he understands that everyone makes mistakes and no one is perfect. He or she doesn't judge you harshly for mistakes you have made.

3. The therapist should have expertise in issues similar to yours and experience working with other people who have those issues.

4. You must be comfortable with the orientation of the therapy.

Some things to know about therapists

1. Therapists are bound by rules of confidentiality. That means they are not allowed to share anything that you say with anyone else. Whatever you say in the therapist's office, stays in the therapist's office. If you ever find out that this confidentiality is being broken, you should stop seeing the therapist and report him or her. It is very important that what you say to your therapist stays private so that you can trust him or her.

2. You should never let the therapist say or do anything that makes you feel unsafe. Touching is not appropriate. Sexual overtures are never appropriate. If the therapist asks to do something with you socially outside of therapy, no matter how flattered you might be, this is not a good idea. Similarly, you shouldn't ask your therapist to do anything with them socially outside of therapy

either. There need to be proper boundaries for therapy to work.

One thing that often happens in therapy is called transference. It basically means that you start feeling a lot of emotions and feelings for your therapist that you are actually feeling towards a significant person in your life, but they get redirected to the therapist because they are there in the moment. You may feel anger towards or even think you feel sexual feelings towards the therapist. It is important the therapist knows how to work appropriately with these feelings and set the proper boundaries so both of you can be safe while doing therapy work.

3. You have the choice to terminate therapy at any time. Don't let a therapist bully you into thinking you need to be there longer than you are comfortable with (say, years, for example). At the same time, try not to run away at the first sign of discomfort as you will never get anywhere that way. It can take a while to build trust and feel like you are making any progress in the therapy process.

4. Therapy takes time. If you expect a change in just a session or two, you will be disappointed. You have to give it time to work and sink in. Change happens gradually, and it can be hard to be patient, but it is necessary. There are some therapists that promise results in just a few sessions, and that can be helpful for some things, but in general to make huge changes in your life, you have to give it time.

Psychotherapy: Experience from the Perspective of a Woman with Asperger's

The first branch of therapy we discussed was psychotherapy or talk therapy. Now, a good therapist may combine a lot of methods together. When you ask their orientation, they will often say they don't have one; they take whatever seems to fit from a variety of disciplines. That is fine, too. Sometimes, it can be hard to separate them. Basically, talk therapy is talking, and cognitive therapy or behavior therapy is more focused on just your thoughts and behaviors and how to change them. The latter is much less emotionally based than the former. It is more about the present and facts and trying to get you to see facts. Psychotherapy or talk therapy can go all over the place—you can talk about your past, your present, your emotions, what you had for breakfast this morning, whatever you want.

Talk therapy

One adult with Asperger's tells how traditional talk therapy helped with some of the issues she was experiencing.

"Therapy Helped Lessen My Anxiety"

One Woman's Story

I didn't know what to expect when I walked in. The woman seemed very friendly and warm, though, and I got a good vibe from her. We talked about the anxiety I was experiencing and my feeling inadequate in social situations. Not knowing what to say, how long to say it for, who to say it to. Not knowing when to start and when to stop. I told about how the anxiety I was experiencing was making me feel obsessive about completing a lot of rituals I felt I needed to do that didn't make much sense and took up a lot of time. And about my depressive thoughts and occasional suicidal thoughts. I also talked about some of the problems I was having with my family not understanding all of my difficulties. How it would take ten times as long for me to do something because I'd have to go back and do it again to make sure it was done right. I just felt like a nervous wreck and didn't even realize I had so many issues until I started talking.

Some people ask me what it was that helped me in therapy. I saw her for about two years or so, every couple weeks. It wasn't any one thing or one technique. I didn't even feel like any techniques were used on me. Nothing fancy that you have to learn in school, I felt. Rather, I felt that she cared. I felt a connection with her. From her face and tone of voice and what she said to me, I had this feeling of empathy from her. And that seemed to loosen all of the fear and anxiety in me. Having this one strong connection to another human being, which I had never had before, made me not so scared of the rest of the world. I started feeling less of a need to perform all of the obsessive rituals I had to do before. I felt a little more relaxed and able to talk to people without worrying so much. It was just like a huge weight had been lifted from me. I didn't have to worry so much.

***

So we can see that the process of simply talking out all of the stressful issues in one's life can have a positive effect. It is not even so much the talking as much as the sense of truly being listened to that can really help the adult with Asperger's, as well as the rest of us, feel more stable and competent in our lives. Sometimes the therapist will give advice and direction as well. Sometimes they will use cognitive exercises to get us to see things in a different way. It takes time and it doesn't happen overnight, but if you give it time you may gradually see a shift in the way you think and experience the world.

Shortcomings of Talk Therapy

Talk therapy can help a lot of people but it is not for everyone. Sometimes, talk therapy can be helpful for people with AS just because they are so glad to have someone who will listen to them. But it won't always help with anxiety or depression problems, or target any other specific things that need help. Nomi Kaim describes this best on her piece printed on the Asperger's Association of New England site (www.aane.org):

"People with AS may thrive on the opportunity for one-on-one conversation provided by the therapeutic interaction, but we often don't benefit much past this happy occasion to be listened to. We don't carry things with us beyond the weekly session. This problem may stem from a difficulty in understanding and applying abstract symbolism and metaphors (though I'm not sure exactly how that would work), or it may arise because people with Asperger's are so verbal we can "talk the talk" without necessarily ever learning to "walk the walk"—both inside and outside of therapy sessions. Or there may be some other reason entirely. If anything is becoming clear in this age of neuropsychology, it is that "just talking about it" doesn't work for everyone."

So where does that leave us? Well, sometimes when just talking about it doesn't work, it's best to take a more hands-on approach.

Cognitive Behavioral Therapy (CBT)

Cognitive behavior therapy, or CBT, is a more direct and hands-on approach to solving your problems. A CBT therapist will ask you about your thoughts, and then try to get you to look at them with a critical viewpoint. The theory behind CBT is that thoughts control and shape behavior. Change your thoughts, and your behavior (and anxiety, depression, worldview, etc) will change, too.

The National Institute of Mental Health, or NAMI, at www.nami.org, describes CBT this way:

"Cognitive-Behavioral Therapy (CBT) is an empirically supported treatment that focuses on patterns of thinking that are maladaptive and the beliefs that underlie such thinking. For example, a person who is depressed may have the belief, "I'm worthless," and a person with a phobia may have the belief, "I am in danger." While the person in distress likely holds such beliefs with great conviction, with a therapist's help, the individual is encouraged to view such beliefs as hypotheses rather than facts and to test out such beliefs by running experiments. Furthermore, those in distress are encouraged to monitor and log thoughts that pop into their minds (called "automatic thoughts") in order to enable them to determine what patterns of biases in thinking may exist and to develop more adaptive alternatives to their thoughts. People who seek CBT can expect their therapist to be active, problem-focused, and goal-directed."

One reason that CBT often works better with adults with AS is that it focuses on the mind. Adults with AS often have highly developed systems of thought and cognition; they just need some guidance sometimes on how to put all this thinking power to good use. They can sometimes be taught how to turn around their thinking so that it is more productive.

CBT operates based on a theory that AS is a neurologically based set of information processing problems. Since adults with AS process information about the world in different ways than typical people, it affects the way they understand the world and learn about the world and themselves. AS is described by some as a "core social disorder" in which information processing problems are at the root of most of the problems one sees in AS. This shows itself in several ways.

Three Information Processing Problems
Associated with AS Adults

1. **Problems processing information about others, also known as social cognition:**

   Lack of ability to imagine what others are thinking or feeling; lack of ability to use nonverbal cues to understand social situations; lack of ability to adapt language for use pragmatically in social situations (such as you know how to use language but can't use it in the way people expect you to in order to fit the social situation well). The way you process information then makes it hard to effectively communicate with other people.

2. **Processing of information about yourself:**

   Many adults with AS have trouble in the ways they perceive themselves and in the way they regulate their emotions. They sometimes either do not know what they are feeling, or feel way too much and don't know what to do with it. Also, people with AS have trouble regulating sensory information that comes in, and usually, again, feel way too little or way too much.

3. **Processing of information that isn't social:**

   Executive functioning is often said to be one of the biggest deficits in adults with AS. Planning, organizing, seeing context, seeing the big picture in things, can all be difficult. People with AS often see things in details and then don't know what to do with the details.

Therefore, we see that social perception and the use of social cues is a very important skill to learn for people with Asperger's. CBT is a directed therapy that can target these deficits. The therapist can walk the adult through examples of social situations, and ask the adult what he or she would think or be doing in any given situation. The therapist can then try to correct any faulty assumptions or social knowledge that comes up in discussing the situation. The client can also take situations from their life to talk about. By talking about what went wrong in each situation, the therapist can help the client with AS see what he or she should be doing next time for a better outcome. He can start to change the way the AS brain is wired and try to make better connections with better information and more knowledge about how to correctly handle various social situations. This in turn means greater social success for the adult with AS, less anxiety and less depression.

The Sandwich Shop

Think of all the social steps involved in even ordering a sandwich in a shop. You have to know where to stand, where the line starts, where the line ends, which way to face, what to say when it's your turn to order, whether or not it's okay to engage in conversation with others while waiting, whether it's okay to move your arms or hands in strange ways. An adult with AS could make an error in judgment in any of these ways and be perceived as rude. The therapist can help the client see that yes, you need to be faced forward and quiet, you need to say X when you want to order, you need to not give your life story to the clerk, and so forth.

A lot of times adults will have anxiety and depression from their disability and differences. A good therapist can help the client see what their strengths are and see that they just have a different way of thinking and processing information. Their different way might cause them some stress and difficulty but they can learn coping mechanisms to better interpret social information. Meanwhile, they shouldn't sell themselves short on all the things they CAN do. They just need to learn more efficient ways to process the huge amounts of information this world gives us. Many different types of therapy can help with this, but CBT in particular has a reputation for being able to change the very way adults with AS think and kind of re-wire them to be able to think in more effective patterns and ways.

Schemas

Schemas represent our self image—how we see ourselves and the world. Sometimes we have negative schemas of ourselves. "I am helpless," "I am not good for anything," "I cannot take care of myself." We might also have schemas for other people that stem from our past experiences with them, but may not be accurate. "I need other people to protect me from bad things happening." or "People can't be trusted." We can also have schemas about the world being an unsafe place, and about the future being dangerous and unpredictable, and about never being normal. These are just some examples of some negative schemas that are common for adults with AS to have. They often stem from past experience but are not always accurate. They affect the adult's ability to be motivated to change things so his future is different than his past. They cause depression and anxiety and lack of will to try to change. A cognitive therapist will examine these thoughts closely with the client.

They will ask for examples of why the client feels that way. Using evidence of examples provided by the client, the therapist will attempt to get the client to see that these schemas are not true. The adult with AS CAN be independent and take care of himself. He is capable and powerful, and here's why. He doesn't need other people to take care of him.

Talking about it can be wonderful but sometimes you need someone who will examine your thoughts very closely and challenge you on them so that you can start on the road to changing them.

Research on CBT and Asperger's has been promising. Many studies have shown that it can reduce anxiety in adults with Asperger's. According to the Autism Speaks website, they have found that:

"People with autism often experience debilitating levels of anxiety, and several presentations investigated the use of cognitive behavioral therapy (CBT) to help them manage their anxiety. CBT is a talk therapy approach that promotes awareness of the items or situations that make a person anxious, encourages a person to think through alternative responses, and coaches him or her on coping strategies. Judy Reaven, Ph.D. (Univ. of Colorado-Denver), presented promising results of a group CBT intervention she adapted for autism. After twelve weeks of meeting with a group of four youths with autism and their parents, 78% of the participants had reduced anxiety, almost twice that found when following standard treatments. Jonathan Weiss, Ph.D. (Haifa Univ.), also presented data showing reductions in anxiety using a group CBT approach specifically designed for adults."

Traditional talk therapy and CBT are both really forms of talk therapy, but one is more focused on thought analysis and changing things directly, while the other is a bit more free flowing.

Social skills / Group Therapy

Another form of therapy that uses a lot of the ideas mentioned above is social skills therapy or groups. The therapist will try to teach the client what went wrong and how to make it right in various social situations. Social groups can be very useful for adults with Asperger's to practice their social skills. To some degree, behavior therapy can still be used in adults with Asperger's, but it will have a lot overlaps with the cognitive therapy we already discussed.

There are other forms of therapy for adults with autism, but these are the two most popular approaches. Most dovetail off of each other. The most important component of therapy for adults with Asperger's is that the adult's presenting issues are understood in a respectful and empathic way, and that the therapist attempts to resolve the issues for the client in a way that feels safe and effective for the client.

Occupational Therapy (OT)

Talk therapy is not the only game in town for adults who are wishing to seek therapy for their issues. Another major form of therapy is called occupational therapy, or OT. One form of OT is called *sensory integration therapy*. Since adults with AS often have many sensory issues, sometimes this kind of therapy can be helpful. If you are an adult with AS and notice that you have trouble with and get overwhelmed in noisy environments, such as buses, the workplace, stores and so on, or if you can't function around certain smells, or can only wear one outfit because you can't stand the feeling of all other clothes; if you jump easily and can't stand chaos, then sensory integration therapy might work for you to help with some of those issues.

All around us, every day, we receive tons of sensory information. People with a normal system will tune out most of the things they do not need to be aware of at any given time. People with sensory issues, though, cannot process or filter out ANYTHING. Everything is too loud, too bright, too tight, too distracting, their nervous system reacts over and over again to all of the sensory stimuli in their environment. There are some techniques a therapist can use to help a person better modulate sensory information that they are receiving.

For example, if you have overly sensitive hearing, one thing a therapist can do is called *auditory integration therapy*. This basically involves having you listen to specially prepared tapes of different tones and frequencies, and special kinds of music that can actually change the way the brain processes auditory information. This will make you less over stimulated by loud noises and such. Headphones are used for this, and usually around twenty or so (the number can vary) half an hour sessions are required before any improvement can be seen. This does not work for everyone, but has been shown to help many.

Another thing that can help people who are sensitive to touch, or have problems with the feeling of clothing, is something called the *Wilbarger Deep Pressure technique*. Basically, the person's skin is brushed in a certain way with a certain type of brush. This helps stimulate certain nerves and receptors in the body and brain, and over time can make you more tolerant to the feeling of certain fabrics and more tolerant of things touching you. It also is supposed to help you mentally organize yourself, and improves mind-body communication. Since many people with AS crave deep pressure, this can help them relax. Generally, this is done every couple of hours for a certain time period, by someone who is trained in the method (most occupational therapists who work with those on the autistic spectrum are).

There are different kinds and sorts of sensory integration therapy. An occupational therapist is usually the person who will carry these out. Sometimes OTs are covered by insurance, but sometimes they aren't, so you will want to check. Sometimes things that are OT activities will look almost look like playing, but they are activities designed to help your sensory and nervous system re-align itself better so that it functions better.

Swings, therapy balls, slides, and ramps are not out of a place in the office of an occupational therapist working on sensory integration.

Depending on whether you are hyposensitive to sensory information, that is, you don't feel it enough, or you are hypersensitive, meaning you feel it too much, the therapist will create different activities for you to do. Swinging, deep pressure activities, jumping on trampolines, climbing walls, balance beams, and playing with squeezable toys, all activate different systems in the brain and body, and the more you use certain systems, the more the brain is rewired to be able to deal with that kind of input—if you do it under a trained therapist who knows what they are doing.

Weighted blankets can be calming to some people; the added weight acts as a pressure to relax the nervous system. The therapist can recommend this and other techniques depending on your unique problems.

Not all occupational therapists have had training in sensory integration techniques, and therapists who have received a lot of training are often very expensive. You should make sure the OT you work with has had training with working with people who have AS and sensory dysfunction before you start.

Other forms of occupational therapy

A lot of times adults with AS need help learning and navigating the basic skills of life. They need help learning how to cook and be safe in the kitchen. They need help learning how to balance a checkbook and navigate their financial life. They might need help learning how to use a bus system, using a telephone, or keeping all of their affairs managed. There are a lot of small details that make up life and are ultimately very important. It is the job of an occupational therapist to assess what a client needs to be better functioning in all areas of their lives, and develop a plan to help them get there. Some OTs work with people who have mobility impairments to help them figure out how to get around their disability and do things like cook and take care of daily household tasks. Really, an OT does anything the person they are working with needs them to do to try to help them achieve the goal of independent living. They help the person find ways to overcome their disability and make plans and systems to function in the world.

Other therapies

Besides psychotherapy and occupational therapy, what else is out there to help adults with Asperger's? There are always plenty of alternative therapies that one can find, but the question always remains if any of them are actually any good or useful. Most have not had enough studies done on them to tell.

One such alternative therapy that some have found useful is *hyperbaric oxygen treatment*. The person is put in a room with a very pure, high percentage of oxygen. The theory is this increases oxygen tissue concentration and increases brain and body function, and many with autism and Asperger's have seem improvement from this.

Some people have seen results from *chiropractic treatments*. Some chiropractors are trained in ways to do adjustments on autistic patients that increase brain and body alignment and function.

Nutrition is of course important as discussed in an earlier chapter. Certain vitamins and supplements, and staying away from certain foods, can improve functioning and mental states by quite a lot. Omega 3s, for one, support brain function and should be added to one's diet as much as possible.

All in all, the most effective therapies for adults with Asperger's are talk therapy, cognitive behavior therapy, and occupational therapy. These therapies can reduce anxiety and depression, help with social skills, and help with sensory issues. All adults who feel like they need some help with some problems in their lives should try to seek out qualified therapists in these fields.

Where can I find a therapist?

The first place to start is usually a referral from your primary doctor. They will often know a good therapist who could be a match for what you are seeking. Another thing is by word of mouth, if you have any friends who can give you advice of local names in town. You can go online to sites like Psychology Today which maintain extensive, searchable lists of different kinds of therapists in most towns in America. Local autism groups might know of some good names; your local Asperger's adult support group will probably be a gold mine. Just ask the other members who they see. Ask parents in a parent group if they've had any success with local therapists. When all else fails, look in the phone book, but make sure to interview the therapist before seeing them. Try to get a feel on the phone if you'd get along with this person. And ask about their orientation for therapy (talk, analytic, cognitive, everything, or whatever) and experience with Asperger's. There are many ways to go about doing this. Just remember, if you don't like the first person you find, you can always try again, as frustrating as that may be.

How do I pay for a therapist?

Many therapists take insurance, but some don't. You need to ask them about this up front. Some will do a sliding scale for those with less ability to pay, and some won't. Usually you are responsible for the co-pay even if the insurance does pay. These fees can differ but the average is around $20 per visit. If you can't find anyone who takes your insurance, there are often community counseling centers that offer low cost therapy. There is no guarantee these counselors will know anything about Asperger's related issues, however.

Scott Davis gave some good advice about paying for therapy at www.findingyourmarbles.com (unfortunately, the website no longer is active). He mentions that many workplaces will have employee assistance programs to help pay for therapy costs of employees:

"Check to see if your employer offers an employee assistance program (EAP). These programs are confidential (your employer won't know that you have used it) and they are generally quite good at providing therapy services. There will be some restrictions, for example you will probably be required to use one of the Program's therapists, and the therapy will be for a limited time (usually 10-12 sessions) but the program is free. Some EAP providers also offer therapy alternatives such as online therapy and phone therapy."

He also notes that some churches will help pay for therapy or offer their own, such as Catholic Family Services. They may also know of organizations that can help pay for or subsidize therapy costs.

So there you have it. The problems you face as an adult ARE manageable with help. You don't have to suffer alone. You can feel better about yourself, have more confidence in your place in the world. You can learn how to interact with people better. You can feel more comfortable in your skin. There are many different kinds of therapies available to you that can help you or your loved one with AS. Remember, never be ashamed that you are getting therapy. More people are in therapy than you can possibly know. A wide range of people find it useful for different things. May this information help start a better future for you and your loved ones.

11. Nutrition and Eating Right

There are many components to a healthy and happy life. Your social life, your emotional health, your job, these are all important. But one thing that a lot of people, those with Asperger's included, often do not think about is their diet. What they eat on a regular basis. They may casually run to McDonald's for a hamburger, or eat crackers for dinner and ice cream for breakfast. They figure as long as it is food it works. Many feel they do not have the time to eat properly, and many do not think it is very important to give much time and thought to what you eat. But eating right is actually a very big component of health. You will feel much happier, content and a sense of well being if your diet matches what your body needs. Your mood can improve, health issues can improve, digestion issues you thought would never go away can disappear overnight. On the right diet, you can see less agitation, less aggression, fewer meltdowns. Did you know that many adults with Asperger's have undiagnosed food intolerances that cause irritability, lack of focus, and other emotional and cognitive problems? Did you know that eating food grown with pesticides can negatively affect your health? In this chapter, we will talk all about how to make healthy food choices.

You may have heard the famous expression, "You are what you eat." It is truer than we think. Nutrition is an important part of health. There are several strategies to improve health for people with Asperger's.

Supplements that Can Help Your Health

Probiotics

Our guts are inhabited by lots of friendly bacteria that keep everything in balance. However, there are many ways that these friendly bacteria can get out of balance and start to bring havoc on our bodies, digestion, and functioning. The use of probiotics as a supplement brings everything back into balance and increases functioning.

According to an article on FoodRenegrade.com that talks about the autism-gut connection, "Imbalanced intestinal flora causes malabsorption of nutrients in the gut. You could be feeding yourself or your children the healthiest foods on the planet, but if your digestion isn't working properly, you will not be well. Rather, the over abundance of bad bacteria in your gut will not only destroy the gut lining, it will also use the nutrients in your food to flourish and produce toxins. These toxins then get absorbed into your blood stream, weakening your immune system, taxing your organs, and throwing multiple body systems out of balance. Furthermore, these toxins can also cross over the blood brain barrier in the right conditions (conditions usually created by the current vaccine schedule in the U.S.)."

The use of antibiotics further throws the flora in our systems off, as it kills both good and bad bacteria. It is highly recommended to start a course of probiotics anytime you need to be on antibiotics. Any health food store can give you advice on the best brands to take. Not all brands of probiotics are created equal. Some have different strengths, some different strains of probiotic.

What are some other reasons someone might take probiotics?

Probiotics can help with bloating and gas issues, and other digestive complaints. Digestive complaints are common with people who are on the autism spectrum, and many adults with Asperger's complain about some digestive malady or another.

EverydayHealth.com talks more about why probiotics can help these health issues: "Probiotics are a new area of digestive health—they're a class of bacteria that are actually good for you (think of them as the opposite of antibiotics, which fight bacteria). By studying animals with gastrointestinal disease and people enrolled in clinical trials, we have learned that probiotics can help people with a variety of digestive problems, including irritable bowel syndrome, flatulence, infectious colitis, and pouchitis, among other conditions. Probiotic use is based on our prior recognition that acidophilus, the bacterium found in cultured yogurt, may have health benefits. While acidophilus does not naturally live within the gut flora (meaning the organisms that live in your digestive system) and is unlikely to provide much in the way of improved gut function, the large intestine contains an abundance of bacteria. Some of these bacteria appear to be gas producing and pro-inflammatory, while others seem to protect against intestinal injury, promote normal bowel movements, and lead to a reduction in gas formation and bloating. The latter category, the protective bacteria, include a number of species, most of which produce lactic acid, a factor that itself may improve intestinal function."

It used to be in past times that we ate a lot of fermented foods that had live cultures in them. Live cultures are full of beneficial bacteria. Miso, yogurt, kefir, sauerkraut and fresh cheese are all examples of fermented foods. Today, most foods are pasteurized, which kills off the beneficial bacteria. So, therefore, we need to work harder to get this good bacteria back into our systems. Yogurt is commonly eaten, but most commercial brands of yogurt are full of sugar and flavoring and have little nutritional value.

Probiotics can help keep away some illness causing bacteria that would cause things like vaginal infections, skin infections, stomach and respiratory infections; it can help fight the bad bacteria off, and in that way is a good thing to take as a preventive measure.

Sources of probiotics

The best source of probiotics is a full spectrum supplement that contains many different strains of probiotics. Again, your doctor or local health food store can advise you. If you don't want to take a pill, or want to get your probiotics in easier to take and remember sources, there are many food products out these days with added probiotics to them. The following is not to endorse any product but merely to provide information about a sample of products that are available. There are many products on the market filling this niche.

Probiotic granola bars

These are granola bars that have a yogurt topping that contains probiotics in them. They are a snack that can be grabbed on the go whenever you are hungry, stored to eat between meetings or after a basketball game. They are convenient and taste great.

Attune is one such company that produces this product; *Attune* bars come in many different flavors, such as wild berry, mango peach, and chocolate peanut butter. *Attune* also makes chocolate bars with probiotics in them, and these come in a wide range of flavors too. Milk chocolate, dark chocolate, mint, even coffee bean, are some flavors that you can get your probiotics in.

Probiotic juice drinks

If you normally drink juice with breakfast in the morning, just substitute your orange juice for the tantalizing flavors of a probiotic juice drinks to get your daily probiotic servings. One such company that produces these is called *Good Belly*; with flavors like Cranberry Watermelon, Mango and Blueberry Acai, breakfast will never be boring. They also come in small, approximately three ounce "shot" sizes, that you can have any time of the day as you're going out the door to get some energy. This size is fortified with a full multivitamin as well as probiotics.

All kinds of products, such as *Odwalla* drinks, orange juice and other beverages are now starting to come out with probiotic enhanced versions. Not all of these products will be as effective; it depends a lot on how they are made, stored, what are used to produce them.

Yogurts have a lot of probiotics naturally, but you have to make sure to get all natural yogurt with no sugar added.

Probiotic powders

Probiotics also sometimes come in powder form that you can mix with water. One brand that has been sometimes controversial but not well known by most is called *Three-Lac*. This is a dietary supplement that contains live lactic acid bacteria. It includes the strains of bacillus coagulans, bacillus subtilis and enterococcus faecali. One interesting thing about *ThreeLac* is that many parents of autistic kids have reported that it helps a lot of their kids' symptoms. One can assume that it might do the same with adults with Asperger's who have either digestion problems or mental/emotional issues that could be connected to digestion, but no studies have been done on the matter to prove it conclusively one way or the other.

We do, however, have some anecdotal evidence from reviews of the product, this time from Amazon.com:

"I have a 4-year old child with autism. She has numerous problems with her intestines—leaky gut, numerous food allergies and yeast problems. We have tried everything to get rid of her yeast but it keeps coming back along with the horrible diarrhea. Dr. Bradstreet suggested we give this a try and it actually works! She looks and feels better and the diarrhea is finally gone! It has only been two weeks since we started but we are thrilled with the results. If you have a child with autism that has gut and yeast problems (and 90% do), this product may work for you."

It seems, then, that there are a wide variety of probiotic products on the market these days. People with autism and Asperger's often suffer a much higher rate of digestion problems, and studies have shown that problems with the gut can also affect the brain. Gut issues can affect concentration, emotional stability, and so on. Probiotics are one thing that have been shown to help with gut issues, and therefore, are an essential part of any adult with Asperger's diet.

Omega 3s

Omega 3s are an essential fatty acid. Your body can't make them but they are essential for your health. Omega 3s help greatly with brain function. They seem to "oil" the gears of the brain. Omega 3s can also help prevent heart disease, cancer and arthritis.

According to the University of Maryland Medical Center, "Extensive research indicates that omega-3 fatty acids reduce inflammation and help prevent risk factors associated with chronic diseases such as heart disease, cancer, and arthritis. These essential fatty acids are highly concentrated in the brain and appear to be particularly important for cognitive (brain memory and performance)

271

and behavioral function. In fact, infants who do not get enough omega-3 fatty acids from their mothers during pregnancy are at risk for developing vision and nerve problems. Symptoms of omega-3 fatty acid deficiency include extreme tiredness (fatigue), poor memory, dry skin, heart problems, mood swings or depression, and poor circulation."

There is another type of fatty acids called Omega 6s. You should take Omega 3s and Omega 6s in balance to each other for the best health results. Omega 3s help prohibit inflammation, and Omega 6s encourage it. You need both for optimal functioning.

Where do you get Omega 3s from?

The best source of Omega 3s are from fish. Salmon is an excellent source of Omega 3s. Fatty fish such as mackerel, trout, herring, sardines, and albacore tuna are also good. Many nuts, such as soybeans, pumpkin seeds and walnuts, have Omega 3s in them, too. Eggs also have omegas in them, particularly ones enhanced for this purpose. Flax seeds and flax seed oil are an easy thing to add to many different foods and a great source of omegas. You can add flax seeds to salads or drizzle flax seed oil on top. Cooking with canola oil is another great way to get your Omega 3s.

You can also get fish oil supplements that have Omega 3s in them.

What other conditions have Omega 3s or other essential fatty acids been shown to help with?

- Osteoporosis: Omega 3s increase bone strength and level of calcium in the body

- Arthritis: Omega 3s reduce inflammation in the body. Reported to reduce stiffness and pain in the body.

272

- Depression: Omega 3s can help nerve cells communicate with each other. Those who eat a diet high in Omega 3s have been shown in some studies to experience less clinical depression than those who don't.

- Bipolar disorder: Studies have shown that those treated with a proper ratio of Omega 3s and 6s showed fewer mood swings.

- Burns: Essential fatty acids have been shown to reduce inflammation and increase healing of wounds.

Many studies are under way to explore the many effects omegas can have on all kinds of illnesses and disorders.

Non-food sources of essential fatty acids

If you are having trouble getting enough omegas in your diet, try a supplement that contains them. There are many different kinds of fish oil capsules out there, but many people do not like them because they can make you burp sometimes and create an unpleasant fishy odor and taste. To solve this problem, consider these two options:

The company *Coromega* makes a delightful tasting Omega paste that contains Omega 3 and 6s. These paste packets have an orange flavor and don't taste fishy at all. You can put it on your food or eat it straight from the packet. You can take one with you when you go so you will have them with you at all times. You can buy these online or at some local stores.

Consider taking oils such as cod liver oil to get your daily amount of essential fatty acids. Cod liver oil has a large amount of both DHA and EHA (the two main kinds of Omegas), as well as Vitamins A and D. Many companies will add an orange or lemon flavor to it to make it taste better. One teaspoon a day can give you many health benefits.

Other Supplements That Can Help

Omega 3s and probiotics are just two of the many nutrients that can help you stay healthy. Some of the others include:

- Vitamin A is found in animal sources, such as eggs, meat, fish, milk, cheese. Studies suggest that this vitamin shows improvements in language, vision, attention and social interaction in some people with autism and Asperger's.

- Vitamin B complex, especially B12: helps brain function, helps to produce neurotransmitters, and can help the absorption of essential nutrients into the body. This can improve nervous system function. All of this helps the person function better overall.

- Melatonin can help you fall asleep naturally.

- Vitamin C can help boost the immune system, and help neutralize free radicals in the body. Free radicals are naturally occurring chemicals that can cause havoc on the body; anti-oxidants such as Vitamin C help control these things before they get out of control.

- Multivitamins are important to take because many adults with autism or Asperger's have deficiencies in a variety of vitamins and minerals.

From the Autism Society of America website, "Malabsorption problems and nutritional deficiencies have been addressed in several as-of-yet unreplicated studies. A few studies suggest that intestinal disorders and chronic gastrointestinal inflammation may reduce the absorption of essential nutrients and cause disruptions in immune and general metabolic functions that are dependent upon these essential vitamins. Other studies have shown that some children on the autism spectrum may have low levels of vitamins A, B1, B3, and B5, as well as biotin, selenium, zinc, and magnesium; while others may have an elevated serum copper to plasma zinc ratio, suggesting that they may benefit by avoiding copper and taking extra zinc to boost their immune system. Other studies have indicated a need for more calcium. There are several laboratories that test for nutritional deficiencies, but many insurance companies will not pay for these tests. Perhaps the most common vitamin supplement used for individuals with ASD is vitamin B, which plays an important role in creating enzymes needed by the brain. In several studies on the use of vitamin B and magnesium (which is needed to make vitamin B effective), almost half of the individuals with autism showed improvement."

So, therefore, supplementation with vitamins you may be deficient in is an important step towards optimal health.

Diet and Food Sensitivities

Vitamins are only half the puzzle in trying to figure out how to achieve your best level of health through diet. People with Asperger's and autism need to be very careful and aware of what they eat and how what they eat is making them feel.

They may be surprised with the results. There are many dietary changes a person can make that can produce surprisingly good results.

Diets

Gluten and Casein Free

A large number of people with Asperger's are sensitive to gluten and casein. Gluten is an ingredient found in a large number of foods, particularly bread, cereal and grains. Almost all pastries and bakery items have gluten in them; pasta does as well. Casein is an ingredient found in most dairy products like milk, ice cream and yogurt. People who are sensitive to these items will have a lot of digestive complaints; bloating and gas are common. Sometimes there will be cognitive and emotional effects such as irritation, lack of ability to focus, spaciness. Removing gluten and casein from a person's diet can often result in huge improvements to health.

From FoodIntol.com, on gluten sensitivity symptoms: "Many people suffer from headaches, mouth ulcers, weight gain or weight loss, poor immunity to disease, and skin problems like dermatitis and eczema. But the common and well-known Gluten intolerance symptoms are gastro-intestinal (diarrhea, flatulence, bloating etc)."

Casein sensitivity symptoms in those with autism spectrum disorders can be different. Wisegeek.com explains: "While in most people, casein is broken down by the digestive system into peptides known as casomorphins, and then further processed into basic amino acids, some evidence suggests that in autistics, this process does not occur fully. The resulting casomorphins, which fail to break down completely, may have an effect on the body similar to that of morphine or other opiates. For this reason, some experts on autism recommend that people suffering from autism avoid casein in their diets."

Behavior problems can result from consuming casein because if you have this sensitivity, it's almost like you are on or addicted to opiates. This is a new area of science that is just starting to be explored.

Susan Bird prepared a fact sheet for the Ontario Adults with Autism group talking about theories of autism and diet. She explained the casein opoid excess theory very well: "The opioid excess theory and the gluten-free casein-free diet provide yet another perspective on the possible link between diet and autism. The theory suggests that peptides derived from gluten and casein, which are normally broken down in the gut and excreted, actually slip through the gut membrane and travel to the nervous system where they interfere with the transmission of nervous signals. The GI membrane in many autistic people has been found to be unusually porous, allowing these peptides entrance into the blood. The gluten proteins found in wheat, oats, barley and rye and the casein proteins found in dairy have opioid activity in the peptide stage when they are not fully broken down. Previous studies have reported some cognitive and behavioral improvements in people with autism after removing gluten and casein from their diet completely. In a study conducted by Whiteley, Rodgers, Savery and Shattock (1999), 22 children with autism and associated spectrum disorders were placed on a gluten-free diet for 5 months and compared with 5 autistic children undergoing a gluten challenge and 6 autistic control subjects. Following three months on the gluten-free diet, improvements were reported in verbal and non-verbal communication, affection seeking, motor skills, awareness of self and environment, attention, calmness, and sleeping patterns. There was less reported aggression. In the gluten challenge group, both parents and teachers agreed that there was a deterioration of verbal and nonverbal communication."

Although most of these studies were done on children with autism, the results are just as relevant to adults with Asperger's trying to figure out how to maximize their health.

If you are avoiding gluten, there is a very large market of gluten free foods available. They do often cost a little more but can be worth it. You can buy gluten free breads, cookies, crackers, and pasta. You can even get gluten free pizza. There is no reason to go without if you have a gluten sensitivity. There are rice chips, rice crackers, rice flour and rice pasta, among other things. Most of these items can be found at local health food stores or ordered online.

The Anti-Candida, Sugar Free Diet

Yeast and candida can be a huge problem for people with autism and Asperger's. Candida is a natural yeast that occurs within the body, however, if it proliferates and grows too large, it can take over the body and all of the healthy micro-organisms in the body. It can make its way into any organ in the body and emit many toxins that can make us ill. Candida can be responsible for a large array of health conditions, such as abdominal gas, fatigue, anxiety, vaginitis, sweet cravings, inability to think straight or concentrate, mood swings, hyperactivity, constipation, acne, depression, learning difficulties, indigestion, poor memory, dizziness, and even sensitivity to fragrances and chemicals. It truly is a scary substance and can cause a frightening amount of conditions. Risk factors for candida include use of birth control, antibiotics, and a diet high in sugar.

According to Dr. Crook of the International Health Foundation, "One way candida may be related to autism is through the disturbance of the normal balance of microorganisms in the intestinal tract. When this occurs, the protective membrane lining the intestines is weakened. As a results, food allergens are absorbed and this may cause adverse reactions in the nervous system."

Since yeast feed off sugar, it is important to try to keep as close to possible of a sugar free diet. Processed or artificial foods are bad for you; try to stick to meat, vegetables, eggs,

278

and yogurt. Pastries or cookies are out. Fruit can even be a problem depending on how bad your yeast problem is, but not as bad as sugary or processed foods. Try to eat whole foods, lots of veggies, and very few things that come from packages or cans.

Organic foods

It is very important to eat organic whenever possible. Eating whole, organic foods will help your body and brain function to the best of their ability. Most of our food supply is sprayed and cultivated with dangerous pesticides that have a great deal of effects when they enter our bloodstream and bodies. Awareness is growing but many people are still not quite understanding of how many chemicals they consume on a daily basis when they don't eat organic.

Sylvia Riley on www.theorganicitalian.com talks about the high number of chemicals that we come into contact with on a daily basis from our food supply.

"It is hardly surprising that chemicals strong enough to kill insects and plant infections can be harmful to the human body and environment. There are literally hundreds of permitted pesticides, insecticides, fungicides, hormones, antibiotics and other chemical additives present in non-organic food, not to mention food additives and flavourings introduced after cultivation and in food processing. All important reasons for eating organic food.

Over 3,000 high-risk toxins are present in the US food supply, which by law are excluded from organic food. These include 73 pesticides classified by the Environmental Protection Agency as potential carcinogens. Pesticides also leak into the water supply—for example, a 1996 study by the Environmental Working Group found 96 per cent of all water samples taken from 748 towns across the US contained the pesticide atrazine.

Toxic metals such as cadmium, lead and mercury enter the food supply through industrial pollution of soil and groundwater and through machinery used in the processing and packaging of foods. For example, lead solder used to seal tin cans imparts residue into the food, despite the adversity to health. Cadmium has links with lung, prostate and testicular cancer and mercury is toxic to brain cells and has been linked to autism and Alzheimer's disease. Heavy metals damage nerve function, block hemoglobin production causing anemia and contribute to lower IQ and diseases such as multiple sclerosis. Organic food safeguard's against toxic metals.

Solvents are also used in commercially processed foods which can damage white blood cells, lowering immune defense. Further, the solvents benzene and toluene, have known links with numerous cancers."

Some foods are better to eat non-organic than others. Safer foods include asparagus, avocados, bananas, broccoli, cauliflower, corn, kiwi, mangoes, onions, papaya, pineapples, and peas. Most but not all of these foods have skins that protect them from the worst of the chemicals. Some of the worst foods to eat non-organic are apples, bell peppers, celery, cherries, grapes, nectarines, peaches, pears, potatoes, raspberries, spinach, and strawberries.

A non-organic apple might look shinier, but that is because it has a wax coating on it to make it look that way. Organic food tastes better because it's more pure. No additives. Organic food takes more work to produce, but it is catching on in popularity. Organic farmers use natural methods of pest control. Organic meat is good because it was not injected with antibiotics or growth hormones that can disrupt your system. Chemicals of any sort compromise your immune system and can put you at risk for many illnesses in the future, so it is better just to not take any chances and eat organic when you can. You don't have to eat all 100% organic, but whatever you can do helps.

Look for a local co-op to shop at; co-ops will often have better prices than large chain stores like Whole Foods, as tempting as they can sometimes be.

Food Intolerances

People have all sorts of food intolerances they might not even be aware of. These can cause symptoms ranging from digestion problems, bloating and gas, to irritability and other problems. The best way to know if you have a food intolerance is to keep a food diary and record what you eat and your symptoms for 48 hours. If you suspect a particular food is the culprit, try doing an elimination diet where one by one you eliminate certain foods from your diet and see if the symptoms clear up. It is also possible to get a blood test to see if you have elevated levels of IgG antibodies in your blood after consuming certain foods.

The Dangers of Fast Food

Fast food is very popular these days. McDonald's, Wendy's, Burger King, Taco Time, what have you...we love our conveniences. We love to be able to go through a drive through in two minutes and grab a burger and fries for just a few bucks. Just like that, the dinner dilemma is solved. No effort, no cooking, no buying of the food to prepare beforehand, no thinking involved. An instant solution to your hunger problem. Available wherever you happen to be at the moment. Fast food is the ultimate in instant gratification. But is it good for you? Is it worth the convenience? You are probably okay going once in a while, but frequent consumption of fast food will really affect your overall health after a while. You will not feel your best when eating fast food; you're more likely to feel depressed or lethargic because you're not getting proper nutrients, or to suffer stomach upset from the ingredients used.

Seven Reasons to Avoid Fast Food

1. Fast food is addictive. Once you start eating it, it is hard to stop. The sugar, caffeine, and oils can send feel good messages to your brain that obscure the damage it is really doing.

2. Fast food is very high in carbohydrates, low in fiber and high in fat. Therefore, it can make you gain a lot of weight quite fast.

3. Many fast foods have lots and lots of artificial flavors, colors and preservatives. These are bad for your body which cannot handle chemicals very well. Our bodies were not meant to consume so many artificial ingredients.

4. High fructose corn syrup, an addictive that is put in soda, has been associated with increased risks of Type II diabetes and heart diseases.

5. Blood pressure is at risk of rising from high sodium content, as is cholesterol levels; these things together put you at higher risk for a stroke.

6. Fast foods have very little nutritional value; you are only eating empty calories that do nothing to nourish your body.

7. If you've ever seen the movie *SuperSize Me*, you will recall how one man ate nothing but McDonald's for a month, and ended up gaining 20 pounds and experiencing severe liver problems.

There are many reasons why you should try to stay away from fast food, and stick to whole foods that you cook yourself and that don't have any artificial ingredients.

For all those reasons and more, it is best to try to refrain from eating at fast food restaurants as much as possible. Once in a while is okay but it is best not to make it a regular habit. The time and money you save will not be worth it in the long run.

Tips for Eating a Healthy Diet

All of this might seem a little overwhelming. You might wonder how you're ever going to have the time, energy and motivation to change your diet in all the right ways in order to improve your health. Here are some tips:

1. **Cook for a friend.** If you live alone, and a lot of adults with Asperger's do, it might not be very motivating to cook for yourself. So try to find people to invite over who you can cook for. It is much easier and more fun to be interested in cooking if you know you are cooking for someone else, too. It can be very gratifying and encouraging to get comments on a meal well done.

2. **Find a diet buddy**. This is not a diet in the traditional sense; you are not trying to lose weight or starve yourself, but merely to eat in a more healthy way. Find someone else who is committed to this too and share notes, meals and recipes. Try to call each other daily to give encouragement and check on each other's progress.

3. **Get Creative.** If there is something you can't eat, get creative in researching alternatives. Spend a lot of time browsing the aisles of a health food store, or research online. Try to find foods that entice and interest you.

4. **Join a group**. Find a group that focuses on healthy eating.

5. **Watch a movie like "Super Size Me"**. Not only will you learn about the negative effects of the fast food industry and but this will motivate you to eat more healthy.

Healthy eating doesn't have to be a chore, it can be fun! You might just discover foods you never knew existed that taste great to you. The more limited you are in your food choices, the less chances you will have of finding the foods you really and truly like. If you take vitamins such as omega 3s, probiotics and a multivitamin, if you try to eat whole, organic foods as much as possible without any additives or artificial ingredients, if you are aware of your food intolerances and avoid things like fast food, you will be well on your way to improved physical and mental health, and a new, healthier outlook on life.